About the Author

John George Schoon, Ph.D., C.Eng. is Emeritus Professor of Civil Engineering, Northeastern University, Boston. His professional experience includes highway and transportation engineering, traffic accident reconstruction, consulting in multi-modal transport for private firms and the United Nations. Academic experience in the United States and Britain involves research and lecturing. As well as numerous reports and technical papers, including those on transport, pedestrian facilities and inclusive mobility, he has published several texts on these topics. Importantly, to the intent and content of this book, he walks, carefully, most days.

The content and views expressed in this book are those of the author only except as noted otherwise.

Pedestrian Traffic

Walking safely –
why we can't and how we may

John Schoon

Copyright © 2019 John Schoon

The moral right of the author has been asserted.

If a copyright citation in this book has inadvertently been omitted,
please contact the publisher who will endeavour to correct this in a future printing.

Apart from any fair dealing for the purposes of research or private study,
or criticism or review, as permitted under the Copyright, Designs and Patents
Act 1988, this publication may only be reproduced, stored or transmitted, in
any form or by any means, with the prior permission in writing of the
publishers and the author, or in the case of reprographic reproduction in accordance with
the terms of licences issued by the Copyright Licensing Agency. Enquiries
concerning reproduction outside those terms should be sent to the publishers.

Matador
9 Priory Business Park,
Wistow Road, Kibworth Beauchamp,
Leicestershire. LE8 0RX
Tel: 0116 279 2299
Email: books@troubador.co.uk
Web: www.troubador.co.uk/matador
Twitter: @matadorbooks

ISBN 978 1789013 474

British Library Cataloguing in Publication Data.
A catalogue record for this book is available from the British Library.

Typeset in 10.5pt Aldine by Troubador Publishing Ltd, Leicester, UK

Matador is an imprint of Troubador Publishing Ltd

Cover design Copyright © 2017 John Schoon

DEDICATION

To all who strive to make our roads safe – drivers, pedestrians, professionals, elected officials and especially to our devoted ambulance crews and medical personnel; heartfelt thanks.

CONTENTS

Acknowledgements	ix
Preface	xi
1 Introduction	1
2 Pedestrian Characteristics	27
3 Design and Education	44
4 Forensic Analysis	59
5 Junctions and Other Crossings	79
6 The Highway Code	106
7 Speed, Alcohol and Inexperience	124
8 Event Data Recording – the Black Box	147
9 Autonomous Emergency Braking	162
10 Vehicle Design Improvements	178
11 Actions for Improvements	190
12 Pedestrian Casualty Reduction Estimates	207
End Note	217

ACKNOWLEDGEMENTS

People's responses to my request to comment on and contribute to the draft of this book are sincerely appreciated, and reflect a key objective in our daily lives. That is, the ability to walk safely to satisfy our needs and preferences – to meet friends, to shop, admire the view, or just get to and from the bus stop. Such needs and actions contribute to the mobility essential to our quality of life.

In particular, Kit Mitchell provided valuable information on pedestrian casualty trends and the general approach to the book's intent; Ann Frye clarified approaches to identifying and providing mobility for disabled people; Ian Campbell offered viewpoints on local pedestrian associations' activities and examples of actual problems; Terence Bendixson addressed wider issues of the book's presentation and my judgement on various points Their comments, however, do not necessarily imply approval of, or agreement with, statements I have made. To my mind, this makes their contributions all the more valuable.

Many others through their publications, actions, and correspondence have contributed to the book. To all of them, many thanks. Of course, any errors or omissions are mine, and I would very much appreciate your telling me about them.

John Schoon
johngschoon@hotmail.com

PREFACE

Jim Perry saw the car suddenly appear around the bend just as he reached the centre of the road. He hesitated, tried to run, despite his 70 years. Tyres screeched. The car passed, slower now, the driver obviously shaken. Jim (a pseudonym but illustrating a frequent event) was in some respects lucky. But this crossing was his and the neighbours' only convenient way to the shops. The reply to his letter of concern to the Council: "….no fatalities have been recorded at this location and so no further action is warranted". And from the town's engineer: "… the road layout is based on drivers' stopping distance and designed in accordance with governmental guidance".

Why were the voice and the expertise of the council unable to respond to Jim's concerns? Why, unlike Jim, are 5,000 less fortunate pedestrians killed or seriously injured in Britain each year? Perhaps not as attention-grabbing in terms of media headlines, this is equivalent to a 400-passenger jumbo jet crash each year with all killed, and another crash each month with all aboard maimed for life. Another 18,000 are 'slightly' injured. And these statistics apply only to the people who walk. Another several million or so are reluctant to walk at all for their daily activities because of their perception, and indeed reality of, the danger – including children going to school and people with even a slight disability.

These figures raise disturbing questions about our organisational, administrative and technical abilities. Some senior highway engineers have observed that the problem is not simply lack of expertise but comes from the public's cultural emphasis on car travel, by their Members of Parliament, policymakers and local authority professionals. They have prompted UK Government reports to employ terms such as "scandal", "cultural bias", "unacceptable", "avoidable", about pedestrian casualties (UK Parliament 2002). Yet the carnage continues. Despite recent improvements over a historically ghastly toll, the UK has:

- the highest rate of killed or seriously injured (KSI) pedestrians in proportion to vehicle occupant casualties of all European countries;
- the likelihood of being KSI 16 times that of a car occupant per mile of travel; and,
- a much lower rate of decrease in casualties than that for motor vehicle occupants since 2005.

A private or commercial organisation having this number of user casualties would be unlikely to survive. Perhaps viewing the product and service to pedestrians similarly would be instructive.

Why are these so-called 'accidents' mostly not truly accidental? Compared to air travel, for example, is our equivalent knowledge of road safety, human factors, vehicle operation, roadway design, crossings, signals so inferior? Or are we responsible for statements in a parliamentary enquiry about pedestrians, such as "… the roadside experience can feel like a punishment" and "Why is the death of a child following abuse taken as evidence of the failure to protect children, whereas a child pedestrian death represents only a failure of a child to stop, look and listen?" (UK Parliament 2002). Is the stated "unconscious or conscious bias of senior officers for car use", even in official manuals not referring to pedestrians as traffic at least partly responsible?

Responsible, that is, for the design, operation and administration of our vehicles, streets and highways, for being aware of only 2% of recent research reports, ignoring pedestrians' time for looking properly before they cross, their dimensions as they cross, or their need to see approaching vehicles soon enough? Is this often inadequate design of infrastructure compounded by unwillingness to mandate installation of pedestrian collision avoidance and mitigation abilities in new vehicles, and a view of the car (Berrymans Lace Mawer 2008) as a potentially dangerous weapon?

The monetary cost alone to the nation in health care for pedestrian casualties is over £3 billion a year – over £1,000 for every family in the country. The damage to the environment when people choose to use their car for many local trips instead of walking is immense. Sarah Sellers, Chief Executive Officer of the Institute of Advanced Motorists (IAM), states: "Pedestrian fatalities are rising faster than any other group right now so it is vital that drivers are more sympathetic and aware of pedestrians when they make their journeys." (Road Safety GB 2016)

At a government enquiry (House of Commons Transport Committee 2009) into road safety and accidents, Professor John Whitelegg likened the use of streets to being terrorised, and that driving and road safety are not regarded as really serious problems. But there is no law or directive which states that pedestrians' 'accidents' are inevitable. The World Health Organization (2013) states:

> Reduction or elimination of the risks faced by pedestrians is an important and achievable policy goal. Proven interventions exist, yet in many locations pedestrian safety does not attract the attention it merits.

Fortunately the carnage has generated much concern. The UK has, by some measures, a relatively 'good' pedestrian casualty rate compared to that of other countries. But preferably, should our objective be to make walking – and travel by other modes – safe, not merely safer, as stated in a recent report (Organisation for Economic and Cultural Development (OECD) 2016)? Is it acceptable to have 5,000 people killed and seriously injured each year and millions discouraged from walking altogether in a country as technologically advanced as the UK? Our society must judge.

This book aims to assist such judgement by looking at how walking can be made safe. We take a new, more detailed look at the needs, tasks and abilities of people crossing roads, including disabled people. This apparently simple task is affected by the current inconsistencies of roadway design, biases and deficiencies of our 'users manual' (i.e. The Highway Code), shortcomings of reporting and accident investigation, and casualties due to excessive speed and alcohol abuse.

Potentially beneficial vehicle technology examined includes the 'black box', automated pedestrian detection and avoidance, the potential for so-called 'driverless' cars, and 'forgiving' vehicle design. The improvements described provide a basis for estimating numerical reductions in pedestrian casualties to get some idea of what may be achievable.

The book is intended for people who have minimal technical background, as well as providing references for people more numerically adept. The scope is intended to assist people who petition their local councillors, MPs and professional staff to develop improved infrastructure and enact legislation to ensure its implementation.

The coverage here is far from comprehensive, given the vast amount of information available and continuing developments in research and practice. *Of key concern, the book emphasises 'on-site' issues and actions which affect our perception of, and ability to, make a specific walking trip conveniently and safely – key bases for determining how many of us walk. Policies, strategies, initiatives and other macro-level considerations, though essential in the wider picture, will be ineffective if we can't cross the road without fear of getting killed.* But a start on walking safely has been made. Hopefully, this book will help – might we say our strides – along the way.

John George Schoon.
Winchester
August 2017
johngschoon@hotmail.com

References

Berrymans Lace Mawer (2008) *Pedestrian Claims.* Motor Claims Update_MGB, PNG, PEN_(RAW, ACH) 11/08.

House of Commons Transport Committee UK (2009) *Ending the Scandal of Complacency: Road Safety Beyond 2010.* Second Special Report of Session 2008-09. London.

Organisation for Economic Cooperation and Development (OECD) (2016) *Zero Road Deaths and Serious Injuries: Leading a Paradigm Shift in Road Safety.* Paris.

UK Parliament (2002) *Walking in Towns and Cities: Whether the Relevant Professionals Have Adequate Skills.* Select Committee on Environment, Transport and Regional Affairs, Eleventh Report. http://www.publications.parliament.uk/pa/cm200001/cmselect/cmenvtra/167/16710.htm. Accessed 5 December 2015.

World Health Organization (WHO) (2013) *Pedestrian safety: a road safety manual for decision-makers and practitioners.* Geneva.

Road Safety GB. http://www.roadsafetygb.org.uk/. Accessed 3 February 2016.

CHAPTER 1

INTRODUCTION

Facts, actions, vision

Why should we be concerned about the nearly 400 pedestrians killed, the 5,000 seriously injured and over 18,000 more casualties annually in recent years? Should we worry about the dangers and intimidation of vehicular traffic, and about the inadequate design of streets, footways and crossings? To attempt answers to these rather obvious questions we start by briefly reviewing the extent of pedestrian accidents, trends and distribution. We examine governmental attempts to reduce accidents and to end the 'scandal of complacency' described in a recent parliamentary report. Future possibilities are then examined through the context of 'Vision Zero' and how this and similar frameworks for reducing the toll may achieve this desirable but – so far – elusive end.

★

Background

Pedestrians come in many sizes and shapes, with a range of abilities and activities. As with other modes of transport, pedestrians are classed as 'traffic' in the 1988 Road Traffic Act (Department for Transport (DfT) 1988. Here is quite a comprehensive definition of a 'pedestrian' given by the World Health Organization (WHO) (2013):

> A **pedestrian** is any person who is travelling by walking for at least part of his or her journey. In addition to the ordinary form of walking, a pedestrian may be using various modifications and aids to walking such as wheelchairs,

motorized scooters, walkers, canes, skateboards, and roller blades. The person may carry items of varying quantities, held in hands, strapped on the back, placed on the head, balanced on the shoulders, or pushed/pulled along. A person is also considered a pedestrian when running, jogging, hiking, or when sitting or lying down in the roadway.

And for the definition of a road traffic crash, WHO states:

A **road traffic crash** is a collision or incident involving at least one road vehicle in motion, on a public road or private road to which the public has right of access, resulting in at least one injured or killed person. Included are: collisions between road vehicles; between road vehicles and pedestrians; between road vehicles and animals or fixed obstacles or with one road vehicle alone. Also included are collisions between road and rail vehicles.

Although often assumed that crashes between pedestrians and vehicles are inevitable, opinions vary. WHO (2013) states that pedestrian collisions, like all road traffic crashes, should not be accepted as inevitable because they are, in fact, both predictable and preventable. Key risk factors for pedestrian road traffic injury are vehicle speed, alcohol use by drivers and pedestrians, lack of safe infrastructure for pedestrians and inadequate visibility of pedestrians. [Author's note: perhaps inadequate visibility of vehicular traffic for pedestrians would be appropriate here also – a matter addressed in later chapters.]

Optimism may be further justified; the UK's House of Commons Transport Committee (2009) states that: "Reduction or elimination of the risks faced by pedestrians is an important and achievable policy goal. [Note the 'achievable'.] Proven interventions exist, yet in many locations pedestrian safety does not attract the attention it merits." Possibly even more encouraging is the statement by the Association of Chief Police Officers (ACPO 2013) – daily and intimately faced with the often horrific implications of road non-safety – that: "However, road deaths and injuries are neither inevitable nor non-preventable. The last few decades have demonstrated how effectively a comprehensive road safety strategy can reduce the number of people killed and injured on the road."

Investigations and solutions for reducing pedestrian casualties continue to proliferate. Government agencies such as the Department for Transport (DfT), Highways England (HE) and, at local level, Transport for London (TfL), and research organisations such as the Transport Research Laboratory (TRL) and Parliamentary Advisory Council for Transport Safety (PACTS) are all continually involved, as are non-governmental organisations such as BRAKE, Living Streets, Royal Society for the Prevention of Accidents (RoSPA), the Chartered Institution of Highways and Transportation (CIHT) and many others.

Yet the killing and maiming continue. Some views on pedestrian safety in the UK are revealing; Professor Whitelegg in response to a government inquiry (House of Commons Transport Committee 2009) stated:

> In response to a comment by Mr Marlow (Select Committee on Transport, Minutes of Evidence, Examination of Witnesses, Question No. 22) stating that Britain was "one of the best in the world" regarding road safety Professor Whitelegg replied: "No, it is not one of the best. What we do in Britain—and government refuses to investigate this properly—is achieve road safety improvements by terrorising people so that they do not use the road. We have the highest rate of schoolchildren being taken to school by car and the lowest rate of walking and cycling. An epidemiologist or a public health specialist will explain this better than I can, but if you remove people from the group at risk – so the population at risk goes down and down – you do not get much of the disease… We terrorise people so that they are afraid to use the streets. The safest

streets in Britain are the most dangerous streets – the busy, busy streets – because nobody in their right mind lets a kid walk or cycle or cross. Elderly people stay at home, worried, upset and ill, because they cannot cross to the post office, which does not exist any more but the street is too busy anyway. We have the lowest levels of use of public space in walking and cycling of most European cities and we claim that is a road safety gain, but it is not."

and, further:

"Driving and road safety is still regarded as not really a serious problem, not really a criminal offence, not really an issue that people should be worried about and should be uptight about; I think we should all be really, really worried and really, really uptight and sort it out. Government has to take a lead…"

The barriers that children and young people face which prevent them from walking to school are revealed in a survey to mark National Walking Month 2011 (Living Streets 2011). Over 2,000 children and young people between the ages of seven and 14 across the UK were surveyed to seek their views on walking to school. The survey showed that, primarily related to transport:

- over a third (36%) are scared about walking to school because of speeding traffic;
- one in five children and young people are concerned about the lack of safe crossing points on their journey to school;
- 62% of primary school children claim to be unable to walk to school as it is too far away, yet government figures show that the majority of families live within a 20-minute walk of the school gates; and,
- 52% of primary school-age respondents are not allowed to walk to school without an adult walking with them. This drops to only 14% of secondary school pupils.

Categories of casualties used in UK statistics are those of "killed" and "injured", defined in Reported Road Casualties Great Britain (RRCGB), Main Results 2007 (DfT 2008) as:

- **Killed**: Human casualties who sustain injuries leading to death less than 30 days after the accident. (This is the usual international definition, adopted by the Vienna Convention in 1968.)

- **Serious injury**: An injury for which a person is detained in hospital as an 'in-patient', injury or any of the following injuries whether or not they are detained in hospital including fractures, concussion, internal injuries, crushings, burns (excluding friction burns), severe cuts, severe general shock requiring medical treatment and injuries causing death 30 or more days after the accident. An injured casualty is recorded as seriously or slightly injured by the police on the basis of information available within a short time of the accident. This generally will not reflect the results of a medical examination, but may be influenced according to whether the casualty is hospitalised or not. Hospitalisation procedures will vary regionally.

- **Slight injury**: An injury of a minor character such as a sprain (including neck whiplash injury), bruise or cut which is not judged to be severe, or slight shock requiring roadside assistance. This definition includes injuries not requiring medical treatment.

The Numbers

Reported Road Casualties Great Britain (RRCGB) 2012 (DfT 2012) states that car occupants make up the largest group of road accident casualties. But there is a marked difference in the distribution of casualties for each road user type between the three separate severities of killed, seriously injured and slightly injured. The three vulnerable road user groups (pedestrians, pedal cyclists and motorcyclists) between them account for almost 50% of all deaths and 60% of all people who are seriously injured.

Recent road accident statistics indicate that in 2015, as shown in Table 1.1, 408 pedestrians were killed and nearly 5,000 seriously injured. More than 18,700 more were slightly injured. This would be equivalent to one large (400 passengers) wide-bodied aircraft crash with no survivors per year and a crash landing of a similar aircraft with multiple injuries monthly. These figures compare with total road casualties of over 1,700 killed and over 24,000 KSI, respectively.

Summary statistics, Great Britain, 2015

	Number			2015 Percentage change over:	
	2010-14 average	2014	2015	2014	2010-14 average
Casualties					
Killed	2,816	1,775	1,730	-3	-39
Killed or seriously injured (KSI)	30,041	24,582	23,874	-3	-21
All casualties	246,050	194,477	186,189	-4	-24
Vehicle traffic (billion vehicle miles) (inc pedal cycles)	313.1	314.3	320.0	2	2
Population (million)	59.2	62.8	63.3	1	7
Pedestrians					
Fatalities	613	446	408	-9	-33
of which: Children (0-15)	57	29	25	-14	-56
Adults (16-59)	301	226	210	-7	-30
Elderly (60+)	253	191	173	-9	-32
Seriously injured	6,145	5,063	4,940	-2	-20
Slightly injured	23,206	19,239	18,713	-3	-19
Total	29,965	24,748	24,061	-3	-20

Table 1.1 Long-term trends and summary statistics, 2015. (Source: Based on Reported Road Accidents Great Britain 2015, Table RAS 40006, Department for Transport 2016)

- Pedestrian fatalities fell by 5% from 2012 to 2013. The overall number of pedestrians killed in 2013 was 35% below the 2005-09 average; the total number of pedestrian KSI casualties was 22% below the 2005-09 average.

- Pedestrians made up around 41% of child casualties and 68% of child KSI casualties. The number of pedestrian KSI casualties fell by 4% to 1,545 in comparison with 2011.

Four main casualty groups have seen a reduction in the fatality rate in 2013 as shown in Figure 1.1. Car occupants have seen the biggest overall improvement in fatality rate, a fall of 70 points in the index for 2005-09, compared with a fall of 45 points to 2013 for pedestrians. Pedal cyclists and motorcyclists saw slower decreases and were around a quarter lower than the 2005-09 average in 2013.

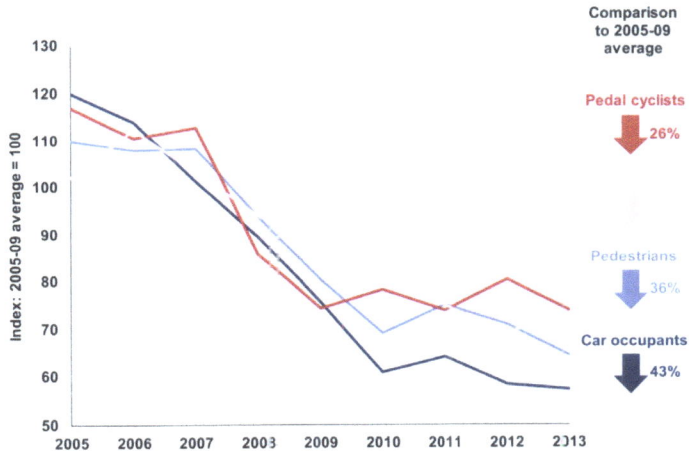

Figure 1.1 Reported killed casualties for the four largest casualty groups, per billion miles travelled (Source: RRCGB 2013, Trends, Chart 7, DfT 2014)

It is noted (RRCGB 2015) that the number of seriously injured pedestrians in 2015 is 2% lower than in 2013. At 4,940 it is still the lowest on record, just under the level set in 2013. Similarly the number of slightly injured casualties decreased by 3% to 18,713, just above the 2013 figure, which was the previous low. Since the number of fatalities has remained much the same since 2010, any changes since then are most likely to result from natural variation and cannot be attributed to underlying causes.

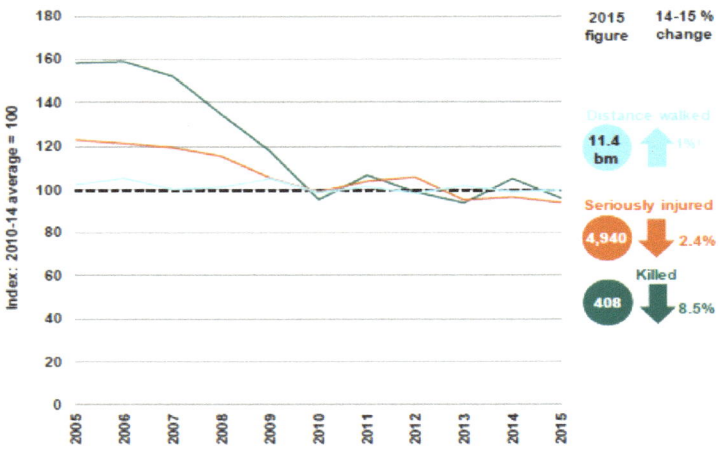

Figure 1.2 Number of killed and serioulsly injured pedestrians compared with the distance walked, 2005 – 2015(Source: RRCGB 2015, Chart 4, DfT 2016)

Although not always directly linked, the number of vehicles on the roads decreases as the economy also declines. This relationship is particularly true for commercial vehicles. Furthermore, there is a relationship (albeit, again not direct) between volumes of traffic and the number of road traffic accidents.

The reduction in casualties during the last few years is undoubtedly encouraging. But the fact that the initial totals were so unacceptably high should make the fact of the recent reductions a mere indication that much more needs to be (and undoubtedly can be) achieved. Recognition of the problem is made in 'A Transport journey to a Healthier Life' (Chartered Institute of Highways and Transportation (CIHT) 2016) which states: "The transport sector is failing to take account of the full health and wellbeing benefits of walking."

Although pedestrian casualties shows a commendable reduction in proportion to the total number of casualties, pedestrian deaths in

Britain as a proportion of all road deaths show the highest values for Western European countries, both for children and for all pedestrians, as shown in Figure 1.3. A valid question, but with no simple answer, is: 'Does this high proportion of pedestrian casualties reflect a bias in the provision of infrastructure, and behaviour of road users, that favours vehicular over pedestrian traffic?'

It must also be noted that the number of reported pedestrian casualties occurred to people who were walking. The number of people who were discouraged from walking because of their perception of the danger or inconvenience involved is hard to estimate. But their numbers are important because a sizable proportion will undoubtedly include the elderly and people with disabilities. Their health and welfare, as well as costly in human terms, also has economic implications resulting from additional medical and care requirements.

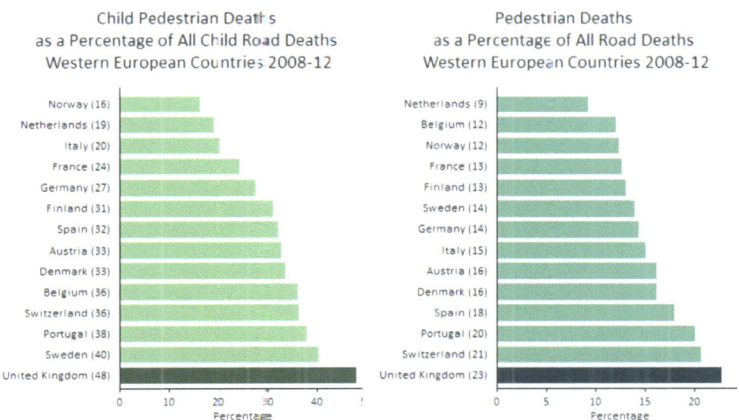

Figure 1.3 Pedestrian deaths as a proportion of all road deaths (Source: Travel Independent Website 2015)

As well as the economy there is evidence that the average traffic speed in free-flow areas and the proportion of drivers exceeding the speed limit have decreased over the last decade. This might not only help drivers to avoid accidents, but also might reduce the severity and number of casualties when they do occur. Technological and engineering improvements to vehicles and highways will have played a similar role in both avoiding accidents and minimising their consequences. Improved education and training will have produced better and safer drivers.

Finally, improvements in trauma care (particularly the creation of major trauma centres in England) will have helped to save lives once an accident has taken place.

The fact that vulnerable road users only account for around 29% of slightly injured casualties might be due to underreporting. Pedal cyclists and pedestrians, especially slightly injured casualties, are both road user groups likely to be underreported in the road accident data collected by the police.

Relative Danger of Accidents

Strikingly, when distance travelled is taken into account, vulnerable road users account for about 95% of KSI casualties. In relative terms pedestrians are roughly 16 times more likely to be killed in a road accident than car occupants. So, if you want to visit the shops two miles away and you have the choice of walking or going by car, you are, statistically speaking, 16 times more likely to be killed if you choose the former. Dreadful though this statistic is, motorcycle users, per mile ridden, are roughly 35 times more likely to be killed in a road traffic accident than car occupants.

Reporting in official documents is inconsistent, with data presented for accidents and casualties without the ability to convert between them. However, certain key characteristics emerge related to pedestrian involvement. Vehicle involvement in pedestrian accidents in 2013 is shown in Table 1.2. Cars and taxis were the greatest source of accidents, with over 3,600 KSI. This was followed by accidents with heavy goods vehicles (HGVs), with a total of over 100 KSI. It is noticeable that accidents with HGVs resulted in a high number being killed (about 45%) relative to KSI.

Vehicle	Killed	Seriously Injured
Single vehicle accidents		
Pedal cycle	2	100
Motorcycle	10	197
Car	212	3,433
Taxi	15	203
Minibus	1	9
Bus or coach	26	193
Van	27	260
HGV	44	105
Mobility scooter	0	5
Other vehicle	10	39
Any vehicle	348	4,551
2 or more vehicle accidents		
All vehicle types	56	349

Table 1.2 Reported accidents by severity and vehicle type (Source: RRCGB 2015 Table RAS10012, DfT 2016)

Major contributory factors, as shown in Table 1.3, were:

- failure to look properly, 58%
- being in a hurry or carelessness, 29%
- failure to properly judge a vehicle's path or speed, 18%.

Pedestrians' alcohol consumption was cited as a contributory cause in approximately 9% of accidents.

Contributory Factor Attributed to Pedestrian	Number	Percent*
Failed to look properly	9,773	58
Careless, reckless or in a hurry	4,871	29
Failed to judge vehicle's path or speed	3,048	18
Crossing road masked by stationary or parked vehicle	2,309	14
Impaired by alcohol	1,517	9
Wrong use of pedestrian facility	1,154	7
Dangerous action in carriageway	858	5
Wearing dark clothing at night	734	4
Disability or illness	461	3
Impaired by drugs (illicit or medicinal)	214	1
Total	16,765	100

* Columns may not add up to 100% as accidents can have more than one contributory factor.

Table 1.3 Reported accidents involving pedestrians with contributory factors, Great Britain, 2015 (Source: RRCGB 2014, Table RAS50004, DfT 2016)

As explained later in the description of pedestrian characteristics it is possible that some of the accidents' reported contributory causes, particularly 'failure to look properly' and 'failure to properly judge a vehicle's speed', may be due to pedestrians not being able to see far enough because of an unsuitable junction design, or other roadway features such as bends, fences, railings and improperly timed traffic signals.

Drink driving is known to be an important factor in all categories of collisions. As shown in Table 1.4, 10 pedestrians were reported killed in drink-driving-related collisions and 80 were seriously injured (estimated at 10% of all accidents due to alcohol use as reported).

Casualty Category	Number
Killed or seriously injured	70
All severities	230

Table 1.4 Reported drink drive accidents by pedestrian involvement, 2014 (Source: Based on RRCGB 2015, Table RAS50001, DfT 2016)

Accidents involving pedestrians in which vehicle speed was also a consideration are not specifically detailed in RRCGB 2013, although it is known that a significant number of such collisions occurred. The number of accidents in which speed was a contributory factor is shown in Table 1.5. In addition, where a contributory factor is given as the pedestrian failing to look properly, if an involved vehicle had been travelling faster than the location and conditions warranted, speed could also have been a contributory factor although not reported as such. See also Chapter 7 for speed-related accidents involving pedestrians.

Contributory factor in accident	Accidents							
	Fatal		Serious		Slight		Total	
	Number	Per cent	Number	Per cent	Number	Per cent	Number	Per cent
Exceeding speed limit	222	15	1,152	7	3,898	4	5,272	5
Travelling too fast for conditions[2]	120	8	1,123	7	5,181	6	6,424	6
Exceeding speed limit or travelling too fast for conditions	342	23	2,275	13	9,079	10	11,696	11
Total number of accidents	1,469	100	17,176	100	89,566	100	108,211	100

Table 1.5 Speed as a contributory factor (Source: RRCGB, 2015, Table RAS50008, DfT 2016)

Actions to Reduce Accidents

Britain's long-term vision is to have the world's safest roads and this will need greater compliance with road safety laws, according to *A Safer Way: Consultation on Making Britain's Roads the Safest in the World* (DfT 2009). This document further states that local authorities must now consider government guidance and determine their own priorities for future targets and investment. Within their new Local Area Agreements, more than one-third of English local highway authorities, such as counties, have chosen to target reduced accidents, learn from recorded collisions, sponsor vehicle design to minimise injuries, co-operate between road safety agencies and other interests, and improve vehicle features such as improved driver vision. Improved learning of lessons from fatal collisions will be crucial – with the power to make recommendations to national and local government regarding:

- improved skills and capacity in local highway authorities;
- highway authorities and the police working increasingly in partnership with others such as educators and the Probation Service;
- good practice sharing among local road safety practitioners; and,
- more effective interventions.

Specifically related to pedestrians a European regulation containing new car and light van requirements to reduce the number of vulnerable road users killed or seriously injured has been agreed by, and with, the European Union institutions. Although the European New Car Assessment Programme (Euro NCAP, www.euroncap.com) has been effective at improving car occupant safety, it has been less effective in improving the safety of other road users such as pedestrians. One reason for this may be that other road users are thought to be potentially anonymous and theoretical to the car buyer, and their safety is therefore likely to be a less important consideration when buying a car. To resolve this anomaly, a major change to the Euro NCAP rating process was supported that will require a minimum level of safety in occupant and pedestrian protection for a vehicle to be awarded an overall star rating. It is believed that this is a major advance and should encourage safer designs affecting vulnerable road users. This is discussed in more detail in later chapters.

Other Euro NCAP initiatives include accident avoidance technologies such as electronic stability control (ESC) in the overall rating scheme. It is hoped that this and other safety features will encourage and reward innovative manufacturers, and hasten introduction of new safety systems into the vehicle fleet.

A further concern being addressed is with HGV drivers' vision. Trends in HGV design have led to drivers having difficulty in seeing cyclists and pedestrians, especially on the passenger side. This blind spot can also be a problem for drivers of left-hand-drive vehicles on British roads. DfT has addressed this issue in the short-term through a programme of issuing 'Fresnel' lenses to drivers of left-hand-drive lorries on entry to the UK. For the longer term, DfT has explored with European partners possible solutions and expects to raise a proposal in the technical forum through the United Nations Economic Commission for Europe (UNECE) in Geneva to amend the mirror standards, extending the required field of view for HGVs.

People who drive for work are over-represented in the casualty statistics. Roadsafe (2014) – sponsored by the Society of Motor Manufacturers and Traders (SMMT) – activities have been to: recruit 'champions' from the business community; identify partners for pilot projects; and engage a wide range of other commercial and road safety interests. Roadsafe has worked closely with DfT and its driving-for-work campaigns, and has developed links with the National Business Travel Network (2008), which is also DfT sponsored.

Although many of the actions taken by the government agencies are directed at motor vehicle drivers, the resulting reduction in collisions necessarily includes those involving pedestrians. The number of pedestrians so affected is difficult to define, but undoubtedly a proportion of the reductions is likely to benefit pedestrians also, and results in terms of pedestrian safety are discussed where available in later chapters.

More concerns to the Government are issues related to methods of recording road traffic injuries, including work-related road casualties; establishing accident reduction targets; funding and establishing independent accident investigation procedures. Details include (House of Commons Transport Committee UK 2009):

- Significant evidence suggests that the current methods of recording road-traffic injuries are flawed. An independent review of the STATS19 system is recommended in order to establish its strengths and weaknesses, bearing in mind recommendations for a British road safety survey. The review should also examine ways to simplify the system, with a view to promoting greater consistency, and consider ways of routinely linking police and hospital data.
- In other concerns the document addresses the need for road safety professionals and accident investigations similar to those adopted for air, marine and rail modes, and for formation of a separate road safety branch to draw together lessons from the fatal accident investigations undertaken by police and other sources.
- It is anomalous that the vast majority of work-related deaths are not examined by the Health and Safety Executive, purely because they occur on the roads. The Government should review the role of the Health and Safety Executive with regard to road safety to ensure that it fulfils its unique role beyond 2010.
- It is recommended that the Government adopts a national target for reducing deaths that is separate from any targets for reducing serious or slight injuries. The Government should also adopt a national target for reducing deaths and serious injuries. This combined target should also be applied at local level where performance monitoring should take account of the inevitable fluctuations in casualties from year to year.

A Vision

A far-reaching, innovative concept, originating and approved by the Swedish parliament in 1997, is Vision Zero (Whitelegg and Haq 2006), the findings of which are summarised here. A key premise is that loss of life is not acceptable. The Vision Zero approach has had a number of positive results but has not gained universal acceptance. It is based on the simple fact that we are human and make mistakes, and that the road system needs to keep us moving but must also protect us.

The vision holds that mobility is crucial for all parts of society. But more traffic means more exposure to potential collisions and associated fatalities and injuries. This is especially so when considering that humans are not made to travel at high speed, and an effective road safety system must always consider human fallibility and frailty.

During the period 1990-2000 there was a 21% reduction in overall road fatalities in OECD countries. While Sweden and the UK have already achieved major reductions in road fatalities since 1990, further reductions have become progressively difficult to achieve (OECD 2002).

Sweden in the mid-1990s set a 10-year target of 50% reduction for 2007. This target was not met; the actual 10-year reduction was 13% to 471 deaths. The target was revised to 50% by 2020 and to 0 deaths by 2050. In 2009 the reduction from 1997 totals was 34.5% to 355 deaths. Sweden's fatality reduction of 39% between 2000 and 2009 was exceeded by reductions in several other countries, such as France, Germany, Spain and Norway (Lie and Tingvall 2012).

Referring specifically to the question put to respondents in the UK (Whitelegg and Haq 2006), "Do you think that the Swedish Vision Zero policy should be adopted as a road safety policy in the UK?", from a sample polled about the desirability of implementing Vision Zero in the UK, 79% were against its adoption versus 21% who supported it. Opinions expressed by the respondents focused on the target being unrealistic, costly to achieve and that life is inherently risky.

Extending the concept of Vision Zero, the report "Zero Road Deaths and Serious Injuries: Leading a Paradigm Shift in Road

Safety" (Organisation for Economic Cooperation and Development (OECD 2016)) may offer guidance on how to reduce road deaths and how a "Safe System" approach to safety can support this goal. The report states that 88 European cities with a population of more than 100,000, including Nottingham with a population of 289,000, have not had any fatalities over a period of a year.

The report highlights four principles for policy and design to achieve a Safe System:
1. People make mistakes that lead to crashes
2. The human body has a known, limited, ability to withstand impact forces
3. There is shared responsibility for safety among those who design, build and operate the system.
4. All parts of the traffic system must be strengthened to multiply the protective effects and ensure that when one part fails the others will provide protection.

The core recommendations to policy makers and the road safety community are:
1. be ambitious – think safe roads, not just safer roads;
2. be resolute – foster a sense of urgency and lead the way;
3. be inclusive – establish shared responsibility for road safety;
4. be concrete – underpin aspirational goals with concrete targets.

Clearly, it is understood that pedestrians and drivers are fallible beings. From removing beer bottle caps to moon landings, human fallibilities are recognized and the means of ensuring the safety of those involved can be devised and implemented. Why not for the safety of pedestrians?

The UK Government in 2014 published its Cycling Delivery Plan with the intention of increasing the levels of cycling and walking in England, yet matters of pedestrian safety are not dealt with specifically and the plan contains no assessment of the gap between the vision and the current facilities for pedestrians. The response from councils that no action will be taken at dangerous crossings because nobody has been injured there is a common one. It reflects a severe imbalance between pedestrians and motorised travel in both funding and safety standards. For example, crash barriers are routinely constructed at high-risk locations on motorways and other fast roads – not just where people have been injured. There seems to be plenty of funding available for high standards to be met for car occupants, but not for pedestrians. Many older people have difficulty walking (or running) fast enough to cross dangerous junctions safely. These people do not need the pilot studies in Age-Friendly Cities (mentioned on page 14 of the Plan) "to create physical and social environments conducive to older people walking". In most cases, it is already clear what measures are needed; the urgent need is fair funding via a fair proportion of the roads budget (Travel Independent 2015).

In line with the achievement of a 'no accident' vision is the notion of driver ability. Apart from the unusual event of inter-pedestrian collisions, and falls due to inadequate maintenance of footways, nearly all pedestrian casualties involve collision with a motor vehicle under the control of a driver. Clearly then, the more capable and careful the driver, the less likely is a collision.

The data cited earlier in this chapter apply to the entire population of drivers in the UK, including the inexperienced, those prone to alcoholism and careless driving, and speeding, as well as average drivers and those more experienced or having special training to improve driving skills. Evidence suggests that the latter group are less likely to be involved in accidents of all types (Institute of Advanced Motorists (IAM) 2011), possibly to the extent of 9% of all accidents. Although detailed data from this source are not directly comparable with national statistics, there is sufficient evidence to indicate a significant improvement due to both a person's interest in becoming a better driver and in the knowledge so gained. Advanced training should (IAM 2011):

- improve skills such as observation and maintaining proper following distance behind other vehicles;

- teach car control and awareness of driving techniques in hazardous conditions;
- support journey planning techniques, including allowing sufficient time to complete a journey safely and planning for the road conditions that will be encountered;
- teach forward planning and awareness of other road users to mitigate the risk of an unexpected hazard occurring (such as the vehicle in front braking suddenly); and
- develop skills and attitudes in deciding how to deal with risk situations.

A telling comment with regard to the vision's ethos of recognising that humans are fallible is that "… training seeks to persuade drivers that even the pedestrian who fails to look properly is something they should be able to manage safely" (IAM 2011). Examples of awareness and improved driving are shown in Figures 1.4 and 1.5 where the driver is aware of, and takes actions to avoid 'unexpected' movements of pedestrians (Police Foundation 2013) and, consequently, there is less probability of a collision.

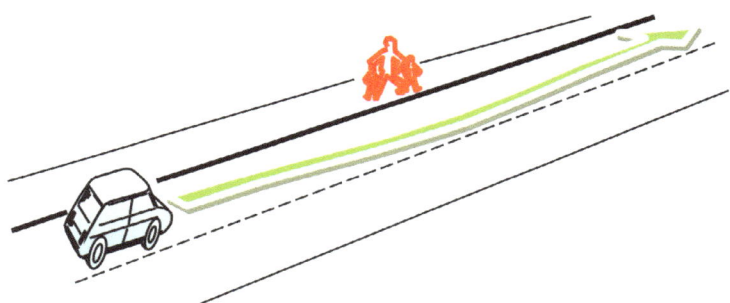

Figure 1.4 Use the brake to reduce speed to enable a safe stop if the children move into the carriageway and take a position towards the centre of the road in case a child steps out (Source: Based on Police Foundation 2013)

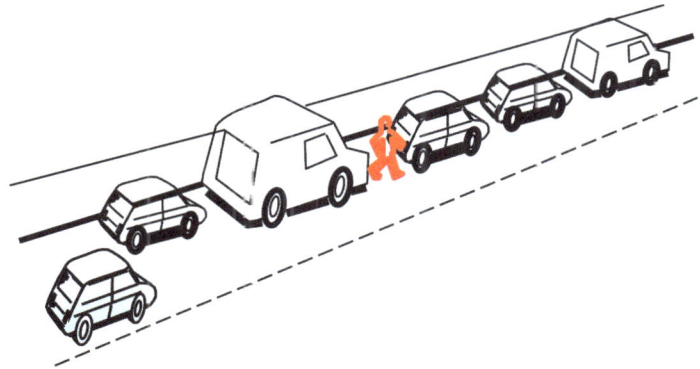

Figure 1.5 Plan for hazards: anticipate, prioritise, decide on action (Source: Based on Police Foundation 2013)

The Future

Regarding pedestrian casualties, estimates based on trends from previous years have been made for future years based on an improvement to the road and traffic environment, per head of population and per unit of traffic (all motor vehicles) (C.G.B Mitchell and R.E. Allsop 2013). The estimates use the Office for National Statistics (ONS) Principal Population Projection and DfT 2013 Traffic Forecast. The projected casualties for seriously injured vary between approximately 2,000 and 3,000, depending on the assumptions for calculation. Because pedestrians killed are approximately 12% of those seriously injured the respective values of KSI must be increased to between 2,240 and 3,360 for the year 2030. These numbers are approximately half of year 2015 casualties – a significant reduction but still unnecessarily high given the potential for significantly greater reductions by year 2030, as detailed in Chapter 12.

Societal Considerations

The public's opinions about the responsibilities of road users for their and others' safety is largely reflected in what is considered 'reasonable'. This is reflected in legal proceedings where a judgement must be made in the case of collisions, and the resulting actions between claimants and defendants. Also, what is considered 'reasonable' is likely to result from societal norms and opinions. An example is where, in the UK, if a child runs unexpectedly from behind a stopped schoolbus and is hit by an approaching car being driven below the speed limit, the driver is usually judged to be only partially at fault. This contrasts with practice in many North American jurisdictions where legislation requires all schoolbuses, when stopped, to display a stop sign and flashing lights to approaching vehicles. Therefore, if any collision between a child and an approaching vehicle occurs the driver of that vehicle is usually held wholly at fault. Shortcomings in data make it unclear the benefits of this law but its very existence reflects a view, very different from that in Britain, about what is considered 'reasonable' in child and driver behaviour.

A summary of legal cases involving pedestrian claims (Berrymans Lace Mawer 2008) includes statements indicating that although a pedestrian has a duty to him- or herself to take care for his or her own safety, it is also noted that a car can do greater damage to a pedestrian than the reverse. Therefore, the destructive disparity should be taken into account in apportioning blameworthiness in a collision and "it is rare for a pedestrian to be found more responsible than a driver unless the pedestrian has moved suddenly into the path of an oncoming vehicle". Furthermore, it is stated that: "The court has consistently imposed upon the drivers of cars a high burden to reflect the fact that the car is potentially a dangerous weapon."

Numerous other cases of collisions between vehicles and pedestrians are indicative of current policy and road users' conduct, the physical characteristics of the road and footway and Highway Code's advice. These are mentioned in the relevant chapters.

Introduction

Prospects for Change

Throughout the chapters which follow there are references to different ways of providing for pedestrians, often involving design changes to crossings and junctions – the places where most collisions between pedestrians and vehicles occur. Making such changes will undoubtedly be costly and will generate opposition due to natural opposition to change. But it is useful to refer to the comments in the *Manual for Streets (MfS 2007)* concerning legislation, the role of Parliament and the courts, and concerns over risk and liability. These comments indicate that there is a tendency among some designers to treat guidance as hard and fast rules because of the mistaken assumption that to do otherwise would be illegal or counter to a stringent policy.

Such approaches tend to restrict innovation, leading to standardised streets with little sense of place or quality. In fact, imaginative and context-specific design that does not rely on conventional standards can achieve high levels of safety. The design of Poundbury in Dorset, for example, did not comply fully with standards and guidance then extant, yet it has few reported accidents. In fact, there is considerable scope for designers and approving authorities to adopt a more flexible approach on many issues. Yet consideration must also be given to the needs and abilities of older and vision-impaired pedestrians for whom consistency, especially associated with crossings, is vital.

Parliament and the courts establish the legal framework for highway and planning authorities and others. The Government develops policies aimed at meeting various objectives which local authorities are asked to follow. It also issues supporting guidance to help authorities implement these policies. Within this overall framework highway and planning authorities have considerable leeway to develop local policies and standards, make technical judgments with regard to how they are applied, including judgements which consider needs and abilities of all pedestrians.

★

> This introduction has attempted to show the current unacceptable state of pedestrian casualties – especially the UK having the highest proportion of pedestrian casualties of all transport modes in Europe and an unnecessarily high number of casualties – together with selected concepts and articulated approaches to improving the safety of walking. The projections of future casualties give some indication of what might be expected if current trends continue. Yet the goals articulated in Vision Zero and the realisation that continuance of these trends is unacceptable should inspire strenuous efforts to greatly reduce pedestrian casualties – and indeed casualties among all road users – now. The chapters which follow outline key issues and ways to do so.

References

Association of Chief Police Officers (2013) *Review of Road Death Investigation, Cleveland Police*. Accessed at http://cleveland.police.uk/get/involved/12629.aspx 08/07/2013.

Berrymans Lace Mawer (2008) *Pedestrian Claims*. Motor Claims Update_MGB, PNG, PEN_(RAW, ACH) 11/08. London.

Chartered Institute of Highways and Transportation (2016) *A Transport journey to a Healthier Life*. London

Department for Transport (1988) *The Road Traffic Act 1988*. Accessed at www.legislation.gov.uk/ukpga/1988/52/contents.

Department for Transport (2007) *Manual for Streets*, Sections 2.5 and 2.6. London.

Department for Transport (2008) *Road Casualties Great Britain, Main Results 2007*. London.

Department for Transport (2009) *A Safer Way: Consultation on Making Britain's Roads the Safest in the World*. London.

Department for Transport (2014) *Reported Road Casualties Great Britain (RRCGB) 2013*. London.

Department for Transport (2015) *Reported Road Casualties Great Britain (RRCGB) 2016*. London.

Department for Transport (2013) *Horizons Programme*. London.

European New Car Assessment Programme. Accessed at www.euroncap.com, 2015.

House of Commons Transport Committee UK (2009) *Ending the Scandal of Complacency: Road Safety Beyond 2010. Second Special Report of Session 2008-09*, p.3. London.

Institute of Advanced Motorists/Tilly (2011) *Social Impact Evaluation using Social Return on Investment*. London.

Lie, Anders and Tingvall, Claes (2012) *Government Status Report, Sweden. Swedish Road Administration*. Oslo.

Mitchell, C.G.B and R.E. Allsop (2013) *Projections of Road Casualties in Great Britain to 2030, for PACTS*, March 2013. London.

Organisation for Economic Cooperation and Development (2016) *Zero Road Deaths and Serious Injuries: Leading a Paradigm Shift in Road Safety*. Paris.

Police Foundation/Stationery Office (2013) *Roadcraft. The Police Driver's Handbook*. London.

Roadsafe (2014) www.roadsafe.com. Accessed 2015.

Travel Independent (2015) Website accessed 15 July 2015

World Health Organization (2013) *Pedestrian safety: a road safety manual for decision-makers and practitioners*. Geneva.

Further reading

Several publications which readers may find helpful are listed below.

Chartered Institute of Highways and Transportation (CIHT) (2015). *Planning for Walking*. London. Provides information including definitions, legal framework and future directions.

Chartered Institute of Highways and Transportation (undated). *Designing for Walking*. CIHT Website accessed 2016.

Davis, Colin J. (2014) *Street Design for all*. Department for Transport et al. London. Addresses design issues including extensive coverage of central area design matters.

CHAPTER 2

PEDESTRIAN CHARACTERISTICS

Abilities and limitations

In the Highway Code's section on stopping distance for vehicles, drivers are shown to require time to think immediately before braking. Oddly, in the design of crossings at important places along a pedestrian's route, no time is allowed for a pedestrian to think and observe immediately before crossing. Other important features of pedestrian characteristics such as a safety margin are also ignored. Pedestrians often complain that there is not enough time to cross. They are often correct. So here we examine pedestrian characteristics not included in the official guidance and how their inclusion could improve the safety and convenience of walking.

★

Drivers' and pedestrians' physical and mental characteristics enable them to get where they want to go. This rather fundamental premise means that designers of the layout and dimensions of roads, streets, crossings and roundabouts must have a clear knowledge of pedestrians' physical and mental characteristics. Yet fundamental knowledge and documentation of pedestrian characteristics is much more limited than that for drivers. Consequently designers, through their official manuals, guidance and procedures, often omit many of the important elements which are essential for safe and convenient walking.

Design assumptions about the abilities of pedestrians when crossing often display a lack of understanding, resulting in pedestrians not being able to see approaching cars until too late to cross safely. These assumptions may be due to the belief that only drivers are reliable and that pedestrians cannot be trusted to take actions to ensure their own safety – understandable, perhaps with young children. Of course, pedestrians and drivers at some time take actions affected by inattention, distraction, illness or other cause, often inadvertent. This is all the more reason why both drivers' and pedestrians' abilities and interactions should be considered simultaneously, but often are not, in the design of crossings, signal timing and other roadway features.

The process that a pedestrian adopts in crossing a carriageway, although typically considered in most official guidance in terms of walking speed only, is much more complex and time consuming. The results of recent studies (Schoon 2010) illustrate this essential aspect of pedestrians' safety and convenience. They show that the mental and physical task of crossing a road involves a person positioning him– or herself on the footway just behind the kerb before crossing and then sequentially:

- observing approaching traffic in accordance with the Green Cross Code of the Highway Code and then consciously deciding to start to cross or wait (all termed the observation-reaction time);
- walking across the carriageway itself;
- gaining the opposite kerb to become fully positioned on the opposite footway; and,
- ensuring that a safety margin exists between gaining the opposite kerb before an oncoming vehicle reaches them.

Key elements of the crossing stages and terminology used are shown in Figure 2.1.

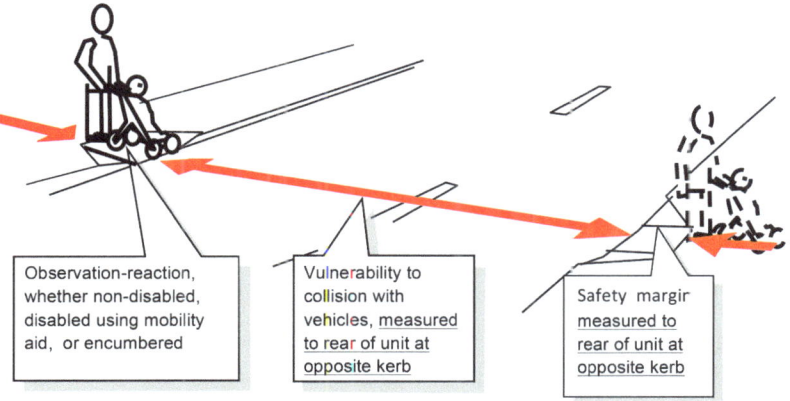

Figure 2.1 Pedestrian's crossing stages (based on Schoon, 2010)

Each of these elements is associated with a time and/or distance. In turn, each time and distance is a key element in a crossing's analysis and design, including estimation of visibility distance to, and speed of, oncoming vehicles and, hence, the layout, dimensions and traffic controls affecting pedestrians.

Typically, pedestrian facilities design is based on surveys of the gaps in traffic that pedestrians have been observed to accept when crossing. But these surveys usually ignore the fact that many of the surveyed pedestrians may have crossed after taking hasty decisions if traffic is heavy and/or moving rapidly. They have also ignored people who are not in the survey because they are reluctant to walk at all, because of the adverse nature of the vehicle traffic. These factors can result in a biased sample and so current estimates of the crossing times often measure the pedestrian's 'time accepted' instead of 'time required'. Here, we look at 'time required', as a necessary pedestrian-orientated approach to determining the actual time needed to cross safely and which should be the numerical basis for designing safe crossing places.

First, before crossing, a pedestrian needs to look around and decide whether it is safe to cross. As with drivers who experience what is called, technically, 'perception-reaction' time (or 'thinking time' in the Highway Code) before taking an action, pedestrians when preparing to cross a carriageway also require time to observe and react to traffic conditions and to take appropriate action, i.e. to look around and start to walk, or not walk, across the carriageway.

The term 'observation-reaction' for pedestrians was coined originally by Schoon (2003) for use with these initial pedestrian actions. The total observation-reaction time is divided into different components. These include the times when a pedestrian is 'blind' to vehicles approaching from specific directions when turning the head to look each way in turn. Observation-reaction is used for pedestrians instead of 'perception-reaction' as for drivers, because whereas a driver in the normal driving task may expect a random appearance (and therefore a need and time to 'perceive' its nature) to be a reason for stopping, a pedestrian before crossing usually expects to see a vehicle, the approximate form and implications of which are usually apparent.

The current basis for signal timing, sight distance measurement and junction design is only on the pedestrian's walking speed and, in the case of traffic signals, a 'comfort time' immediately before starting to cross. However, a more detailed description of the time a pedestrian needs for the total crossing process is essential in adequately designing these facilities to accommodate pedestrians' characteristics. The time required may be broken down into the steps advised in the Green Cross Code. A summary of pedestrians' actions when following the Code in preparing to cross a straight length of carriageway (formerly the 'kerb drill' to stand at the kerb, look right, look left, look right again and, if nothing is coming, walk straight across the road), shown diagrammatically in Figure 2.2, is as follows:

1. First look to the right, approximately 90 degrees.
2. Focus to the right (starts at completion of look to the right).
3. First look to the left, approximately 180 degrees (starts at completion of focusing right).

Pedestrian Characteristics

4. Focus to the left (starts at completion of look to the left).
5. Second look to the right, approximately 180 degrees (starts at completion of focus to left).
6. Focus to the right (starts at completion of second look to the right).
7. Look to the 'ahead' position, approximately 90 degrees, i.e. looking straight across the carriageway.
8. Focus to the 'ahead' position (starts at completion of looking ahead).
9. Start to move ahead directly across the carriageway (starts at completion of focusing ahead and represents the start of the reaction stage of the process).
10. Front of pedestrian (or wheelchair or child's buggy) just enters carriageway and becomes vulnerable to collision from this point on.

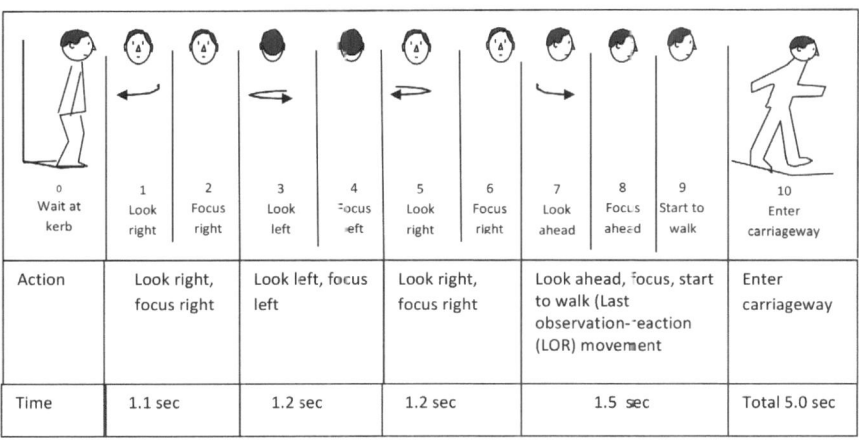

	0 Wait at kerb	1 Look right	2 Focus right	3 Look left	4 Focus left	5 Look right	6 Focus right	7 Look ahead	8 Focus ahead	9 Start to walk	10 Enter carriageway
Action		Look right, focus right		Look left, focus left		Look right, focus right		Look ahead, focus, start to walk (Last observation-reaction (LOR) movement)			Enter carriageway
Time		1.1 sec		1.2 sec		1.2 sec		1.5 sec			Total 5.0 sec

Figure 2.2 Pedestrian's vision and focus process in preparing to cross – the observation-reaction process, using illustrative action times

In this procedure the eyes focus after each head movement to the left or right. While some people may consider the focus unnecessary if nothing is detected approaching, often a vehicle must be judged for its speed and, in poor visibility, a longer look may be necessary.

A fully fit person with acceptable eyesight can usually complete this observation-reaction in about 3 sec.

However, for people who may not be able to turn their heads so quickly, or in conditions when vehicles may be approaching in poor weather, it has been shown that the process can take up to 5 sec or more to determine if a safe crossing can be started. For a person in a wheelchair or with a pram and/or small children it can take considerably longer. The tabulation outlines the directions in which the person would look during each element of the Green Cross Code. It shows that during a portion of the observation process, there is no vision in a specific direction, thus emphasising the fact that focusing can only be done in one direction at a time.

After stepping from the kerb, a pedestrian's walking speed, together with the width of the carriageway and the length of the crossing unit, determines the amount of time the pedestrian is in the carriageway and thus vulnerable to collision with vehicles. Official guidance states that a walking speed of 1.2 metres per second (m/sec) is appropriate for signalled crossings, and guidance related to disabled people on inclusive design may be as low as 0.8 m/sec.

The use of only the walking speed to estimate the time the pedestrian is in the carriageway does not give an adequate actual time required. This is because official guidance for estimating crossing time assumes an infinitely thin person or persons crossing together. However, in cases where a wheelchair is being pushed by someone, or a person is crossing with a buggy, pram and small children, the crossing units have significant length, which may be as much as 2 m. Even a single person will measure approximately 1 m from front to back when striding. Because of this the rear of this unit can be several seconds behind the currently estimated point of movement when reaching the far kerb. For example, if the assumed walking speed is 1 m/sec and the unit is 2 m long, an additional 2 sec (for a car moving at 20 mph this represents 60 ft or nearly 17 m) should be added to the crossing time in order to account for the length of the crossing unit. Also, for a person pushing a pram or buggy or using a wheelchair, even a dropped kerb may have a 'lip' at the gutter, necessitating a pause when gaining the opposite footway.

Finally, is it desirable to reach the far kerb just as a vehicle passes by? Not many people would appreciate this. At completion of the crossing, so that pedestrians should not feel intimidated by having to cross just in time to avoid an oncoming vehicle, a safety margin of several seconds would seem appropriate. This safety margin is never included in current pedestrian facilities design guidance. From observations of pedestrians crossing a typical carriageway as vehicles approach, it would seem that most pedestrians need at least a 2-sec interval between the time when they reach the kerb after crossing to when an approaching vehicle passes that point.

The basis for current design estimates of pedestrians' crossing time compared to actual time, using example times and speeds, is shown in Figure 2.3. Current design guidance (Figure 2.3(a)) is based upon the time taken by an infinitely thin, imaginary person (or crossing unit) crossing from kerb to kerb. But in reality the actual total crossing time needed is as shown in Figures 2.3(b) and (c). To the distance from the point when the person starts to cross must be added the length of the crossing unit and the distance that the unit occupies on the starting footpath and a safety margin at the opposite kerb. Because these two distances can add up to 4 m, this adds significant additional time (approximately 4 sec in the example) compared to current methods of calculating crossing time, without even considering a safety margin when the pedestrian needs to have reached the far kerb ahead of an approaching vehicle.

PEDESTRIAN TRAFFIC

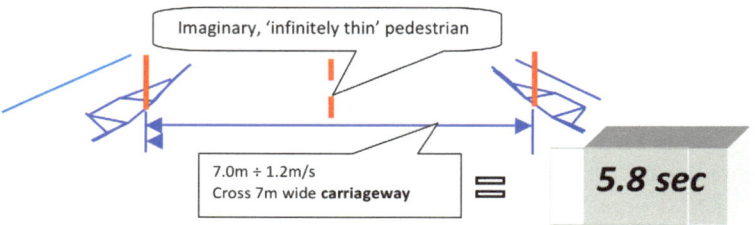

(a) Current official method of estimating a pedestrian's crossing time, i.e. single imaginary point moving only between kerbs, walking speed 1.2 m/sec.

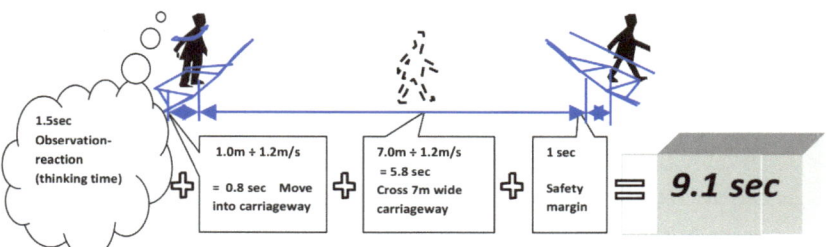

(b) Actual pedestrian's crossing time, including pedestrian's observation-reaction time, length of crossing unit, crossing time between kerbs at 1.2 m/s, and safety margin.

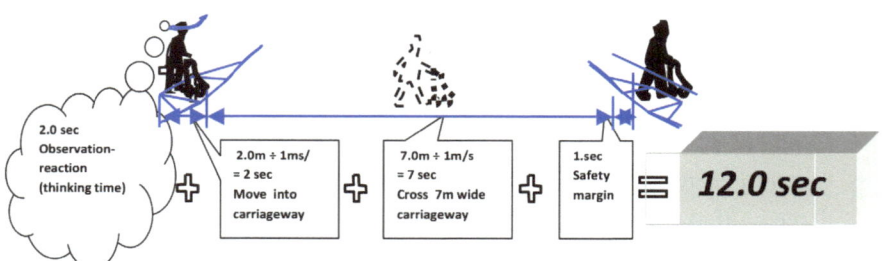

(c) Similar to (b) but with pram or mobility aid and slower walking speed of 1.0 m/sec instead of 1.2 m/sec.

Figure 2.3 Example comparison of crossing times using current design crossing assumptions vs actual values

The frequent complaint that pedestrian signal 'green times' are too short has much justification! Incidentally, in the 4 sec mentioned above, a vehicle travelling at 20 mph covers a distance of 120 ft, or nearly 40 m – nearly the width of a football pitch! The typical times and distances illustrated indicate that the time taken for a person with a pram crossing a 7 m-wide carriageway can be almost double the time estimated using current official guidance.

A further consideration at many signalised crossings is that the post and pedestrian's actuation button is placed a metre or more behind the kerb . This requires the pedestrian to stand at least this distance behind the kerb to actuate and read the sign, so adding to the total crossing time.

Pedestrian walking speeds sometimes lower than 0.8 m/sec, for elderly or disabled people, have been documented in a review (Crabtree, M. et al. 2014) for the organisation Living Streets. The review, which addresses the timing of pedestrian signals, calculates the total pedestrian crossing time in accordance with Department for Transport (DfT) advice based on a 'comfort time' of 3 sec, the width of the carriageway and the walking speed. Several points mentioned earlier in this chapter which would make this 'comfort time' more appropriate for a safe crossing, include:

- a longer 'comfort time' for the pedestrian to look all around in accordance with the Green Cross Code after the 'green man' has started (many pedestrian casualties have occurred because of vehicles not stopping at signalled crossings);
- consideration of the length of the crossing unit such as a wheelchair, or wheelchair with attendant, or an adult with a pushchair;
- a slowing at the far kerb in order to overcome a 'lip' at the kerb and to avoid other pedestrians; and,
- a safety margin, as adopted in any interaction of entities likely to collide and for which the calculation method involves approximations.

All of the above are essential aspects of a safe and comfortable crossing and would seem appropriate for inclusion in current practice.

Summarising the above points, although current methods of estimating a pedestrian's crossing time uses only the walking speed in the carriageway (i.e. from kerb to kerb), in actuality the pedestrian's crossing time needs to include:

- the observation-reaction time before walking;
- the walking speed;
- the length of the crossing unit[1];
- a safety margin; and,
- the official 'comfort time' if several people are waiting to cross at a signalled crossing or where space causes delay due to congestion.

As a further example of the difference in required time between officially defined methods and those if the real characteristics of pedestrians were to be included, consider a carriageway of 7 m width, an observation-reaction time of 1.5 sec, a safety margin of 1 sec and a length of crossing unit of 1.5 m. The difference in total crossing time using the elements of crossing noted above and current guidance would be as shown in Table 2.1. It can be seen that an additional 3.8 sec would be required for pedestrians to cross if vehicles were approaching at 20 mph (30 ft/sec). The implications for this are that a pedestrian would have to see an additional distance of approximately 110 ft (30 m) to the approaching vehicles to that officially estimated in order to cross safely. Alternatively, given suitable athletic prowess, pedestrians could run across, but as most would agree, this would be inadvisable or impossible, as well as being contrary to the Highway Code's instructions.

---

1 A 'crossing unit' would be a single person, or combination such as a person pushing a wheelchair.

Time (sec) \ Method	Observation reaction, LOR (see Fig 2.2)	Crossing the carriageway (7 m ÷ 1.2 m/sec)	Length of unit (1.5 m ÷ 1.2 m/sec)	Safety margin (sec)	Total crossing time (sec)
Current guidance	0	5.8	0	0	5.8
Actual total time requirement	1.5	5.8	1.3	1.0	9.6
Difference	1.5	0	1.3	1.0	3.8

Table 2.1 Comparison of differing calculations between actual conditions and current guidance for a pedestrian's total crossing time

In general official design analysis and practice there appears to be a lack of appreciation for the various components of the crossing process. For example, consider the following statement (TRL Ltd 2006):

> It is known that walking speeds can be affected considerably by the age of the pedestrian, whether s/he is encumbered by carrying a heavy object or accompanying a child, or whether s/he has disability. The time taken to cross the road will also be affected by its width.

In this statement there is no indication that the effective time taken to cross the road will also be affected considerably by the additional elements mentioned above, i.e. the observation-reaction time, the length of the crossing unit and the safety margin, as well as the walking speed.

So far no mention has been made of the pedestrian's head movement and observations during the walking portion of the total crossing process. Although such movement is considered important from a safety point of view, in practice if a pedestrian suddenly sees a previously undetected vehicle approaching, the likelihood of that pedestrian stopping and reversing direction in order to avoid a collision is probably slight at best. It would seem prudent, therefore, to exclude such an action in any analysis and design of pedestrian crossings. Full consideration of the nature, extent and circumstances of the pedestrian's avoidance actions after leaving the kerb is important and can be complex, and considerably more research is needed to adequately document it.

The matter of a pedestrian starting to cross after looking carefully and not having sufficient sight distance to approaching traffic due, in this case, to the presence of an adjoining bend in the road, is documented in the judgement cited by Berrymans Lace Mawer (2008) in a case where "… the pedestrian, who was killed in the accident, was crossing a road near a bend when he was in collision with a motorcycle. It was agreed that this was a safe place to cross and when the claimant started off, *the road was clear*. The motorcyclist should have anticipated possible obstacles when negotiating the bend in the road and should have reduced his speed accordingly."

The key points outlined in this chapter are listed in Table 2.2. These indicate for each analysis feature the current approaches described in design manuals and guidance, the potential improvements in designing for pedestrians and comments related to future design policy. The comments recognise that pedestrians' behaviour, particularly if disabled or encumbered, warrants a detailed approach when analysing and designing the geometric and operational characteristics of highways and streets – a level of detail at least that given to driver and vehicular movement. In this regard, the issues discussed complement existing policies on geometric design of highways and streets.

Analysis and Design Feature	Current Approach	Potential Improvements	Comments
Green Cross Code or similar instructions for users to encourage a safe crossing	Reference to the Code and related functional design requirements are not explicitly described	Integrate the Code with the observation-reaction time before crossing. Reconsider implications for design of the Code's "look all around" instruction	Consistency between instructions to pedestrians and design functionality should improve responsiveness of design to pedestrians' abilities and actions
Location of pedestrian's viewpoint relative to kerb	Assumed to be immediately behind kerb, according to Green Cross Code	For a person pushing a wheelchair or buggy, the viewpoint will be some distance behind the kerb – possibly up to 2 m (6.6 ft)	Sight lines to approaching vehicles are likely to be inadequate if viewpoint is not considered
Observation-reaction time	May be included as 'start-up time' but often not included	Often may comprise a considerable time, especially for people with torso, neck and head movement disabilities	Time to observe and react to traffic may result in increased total pedestrian crossing time
Travel time across carriageway	Normally included	Particular attention to movement speeds of disabled	Lack of adequate time to cross will increase danger and inhibit use of facilities

Analysis and Design Feature	Current Approach	Potential Improvements	Comments
Inclusion of time due to longitudinal dimension of a unit comprising people and equipment crossing	Not included	Adding the time taken for the length of the crossing unit to pass a given point recognises the greater time taken to cross	May be a considerable portion of additional time due to front-to-back dimension of the crossing unit
Instructions in the Highway Code for pedestrians to look all around when crossing	Not included in analysis and design, but implies that pedestrian can effectively stop and reverse direction to safety	Analysis and design of crossing should preferably assume that people do not look around after leaving the kerb, even if they may do so if able	For most disabled people, looking around can be difficult or impossible – as with potentially reversing direction
Time for mounting opposite footway	Not included	Often may be required and may require up to 2 sec or more	If time is required it should be added to the total crossing time
Safety margin time	Not included	A desirable feature of crossings	Pedestrians can be inhibited by 'near misses'
Length of crossing unit	Not included	May add significantly to the total time for the unit to clear the crossing	Consideration should be given to including the necessary time in the total crossing time

Table 2.2 Summary of issues and considerations related to design policy for pedestrians

Keeping in mind the specific characteristics of pedestrians mentioned earlier, and when examining the extent of research and resulting numerical values of road user characteristics, it is evident that drivers are the subject of far more attention. Key areas where all road users' characteristics are of importance include eye tracking and head movement, and speed, acceleration and deceleration. All of these characteristics assist in defining how a vehicle or pedestrian will move and, hence, are essential inputs to the design of highway facilities. Eye tracking, for example the speed of eye direction and focusing, enables the estimate of reaction time responding to events, and peripheral vision angle defines the angle at which objects may be discerned, including approaching vehicles and pedestrians.

Head movement is a determinant of the extent of angular vision which enables adequate horizontal and vertical field of view and the scanning of a particular scene or, more specifically, vehicles or objects approaching from different directions at the same time. Speed of angular head movement is important also. This is because at junctions, for example, vehicles approaching from different directions and constantly changing position, must be swiftly identified in order to enable safe acceleration, braking or steering to be carried out or, in the case of pedestrians, to decide whether to start crossing or to wait.

All of the above characteristics are documented and in official guidance for drivers and motor vehicles, but only walking speed is used in official guidance when designing crossings and other movements by pedestrians. This fact is particularly relevant for forensic analysis (see also Chapter 4) and to junction and crossing design (see also Chapter 5) because the principal cited causes of collisions are "driver/rider failed to look properly", recorded in around 26% of fatal, 36% of serious and 43% of slight pedestrian casualties respectively (RRCGB 2013). Since the avoidance of any collision with a pedestrian includes action by both driver and pedestrian, it is therefore vital that pedestrians' abilities are adequately understood and included in relevant design materials and procedures.

Of considerable importance when considering pedestrians' abilities are the approximately 16 % of the population whose abilities reflect longer times for their actions when crossing. Physical movement, such as head and shoulder movement when observing in different directions, lower walking speeds, impaired vision and hearing are all features which often discourage or prevent people from walking because their routes to essential services involve crossings which are actually, or percieived to be, unsafe.

★

> One of the most often cited complaints of pedestrians is that they don't have enough time to cross safely. The points presented and discussed in this chapter indicate how recent research addresses reasons for this problem. The remedy appears to be a reconsideration of design practices to enable pedestrians, including those in some way disabled or encumbered, to cross safely. In particular, the detailed consideration of pedestrians' capabilities when crossing must be made instead of assuming merely a single infinitely thin entity moving between kerbs, as with current official design guidance. Consideration must be given to pedestrians' times to look and focus in multiple directions; require up to 2 m length occupying the footway and carriageway; cross at a realistic walking speed; and include a safety margin. The points mentioned in this chapter will be revisited in ensuing chapters particularly when addressing forensic analysis of collisions, design of junctions and crossings, and the Highway Code.

References

Berrymans Lace Mawer (2008) *Pedestrian Claims.* Motor Claims Update_MGB, PNG, PEN_(RAW, ACH) 11/08.

Crabtree, M., Lodge, C., Emmerson, P. (2014) *A Review of Pedestrian Walking Speeds and Time to Cross the Road*. TRL for Living Streets. London.

Department for Transport (2005) *Traffic Advisory Leaflet 5/05: Pedestrian Facilities at Signal-Controlled Junctions*. London.

Department for Transport (2013) *Recorded Road Casualties in Great Britain (RRCGB)* 2013. London.

Martin, A. (2006) TRL Ltd Report No. PPR 241, *Factors Affecting Pedestrian Safety: A Literature Review, p.i)*, prepared for Ben Johnson, London Safety Unit, Transport for London.

Schoon, J.G. (2003) *Pedestrian Observation-reaction Times: Concepts and Pilot Study. In Proceedings*: 35th Annual Meeting of the Universities' Transport Study Group, *Loughborough University UK, 2003*. Loughborough.

Schoon, John G. (2010) *Pedestrian Facilities: Engineering and Geometric Design*. Thomas Telford, London.

CHAPTER 3

DESIGN AND EDUCATION

Response to road users' needs

The technical skills underlying street and road design as formulated by engineers, designers and planners should provide the basis for safe interaction of pedestrians and vehicles. Here, we look at examples of how the emphasis on motor vehicles has affected key features of the pedestrian's environment. Highlighted are some ways in which engineers and planners have responded to societal, cultural and resulting governmental emphasis – designs which enable us to walk, often be inconvenienced when doing so and, too often, be killed or injured.

★

The Motor Vehicle Emphasis

Throughout the provision of roads and streets since the private car gained in popularity in the last century a fundamental assumption is that movement by car should be encouraged and enabled wherever possible. Official guidance to road designers states that "pedestrian facilities should be provided to the extent that vehicular traffic capacity shall not be unduly compromised". Section 16 of the Traffic Management Act 2004 (UK Government 2004) emphasises the "expeditious" movement of traffic (meaning motorised traffic), and "the efficient use of the network and the avoidance, elimination or reduction of road congestion or other disruption to the movement of traffic on their road network or a road network for which another authority is the traffic authority". Official guidance on calculating the benefit/cost of new or improved road schemes does not include consideration of non-motorised traffic – even for schemes where a lot of pedestrian traffic can be expected.

The underlying assumption of vehicle emphasis has pre-ordained key features of any detailed, engineering-related design of roads and footways, crossings and related features of the road system. It implies that vehicles should be enabled to travel as fast as the system will allow, having regard to controllability of the vehicle. More recently, somewhat grudgingly spurred by more vulnerable and environmentally conscious people, this emphasis may be changing; we increasingly recognise the drastic toll on human life, financial and economic impacts and gross violation of some of the tenets of civilised life: and, equal opportunity and mobility for all.

Designing for motor vehicles takes many forms. An example of how vehicles are favoured at the expense of pedestrians is where large radii on street corners, as shown in Figure 3.1, enable vehicles to turn faster and so not impede traffic approaching from the opposite directions. Design guidance states that these large radii give drivers a better view of the road ahead and of pedestrians who may be waiting to cross. But nothing is said about the pedestrian waiting to cross safely being able to see the speeding vehicle with a driver distracted by using a mobile phone, and having a much greater distance to cross, away from his/her desire line, exposed and intimidated by fast-moving vehicles approaching from several directions at once.

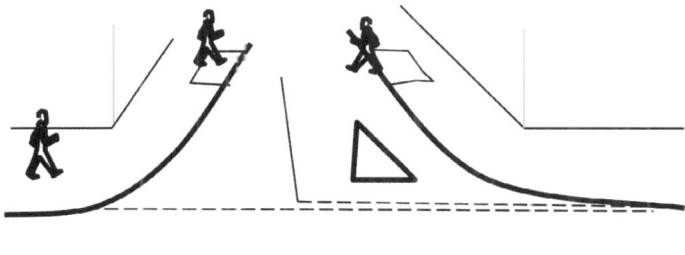

Figure 3.1 Long radii junctions – a long way to walk and faster-moving vehicles

Many places where pedestrians must cross, particularly at junctions, and often defined by the position of dropped kerbs, are where the alignment of the pedestrians' crossing is back from the line of the major road, thereby often obscuring the view, or sight line, to approaching vehicles.

Where the Highway Code may state that pedestrians have priority over vehicles at a crossing, pedestrians often have to cross behind waiting vehicles, and the road markings emphasise this. In order that vehicles can turn at these corners unimpeded, barriers may be erected to prevent pedestrians from crossing, "for their own safety", thereby requiring them to walk further. The barrier may also obstruct pedestrians' view of oncoming traffic, particularly disabled people in wheelchairs and children, both of whose eye levels may be lower than the height of the barrier. Figure 3.2 shows some of these features, including:

- pedestrians' desire line disrupted – difficulties especially for wheelchair, pushchair and mobility scooter users; and,
- difficulties of drivers to see pedestrians obscured by turning and waiting vehicles.

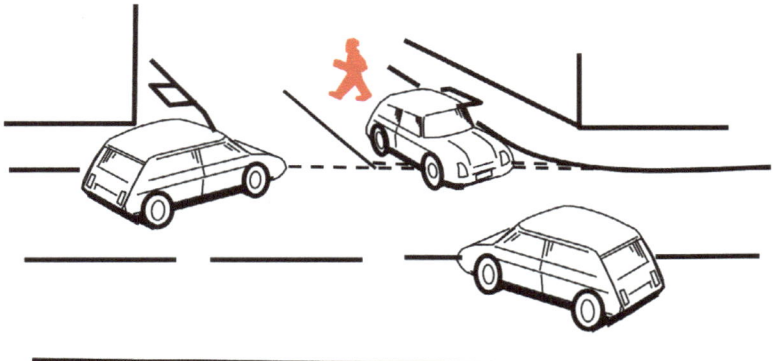

Figure 3.2 Crossings back from major road at junction – pedestrian obscured

Roundabouts are clearly also designed primarily for vehicle use, as shown in Figure 3.3. Their advantages for vehicles again occur at the expense of pedestrians. High vehicle speeds due to large radii and pedestrian crossing locations where vehicle drivers are often concentrating on approaching vehicles rather than on the pedestrians crossing are common. A brief review of published recommendations for drivers approaching and negotiating roundabouts indicates that out of six sources only one mentioned the need to "be aware of" pedestrians about to cross or actually crossing.

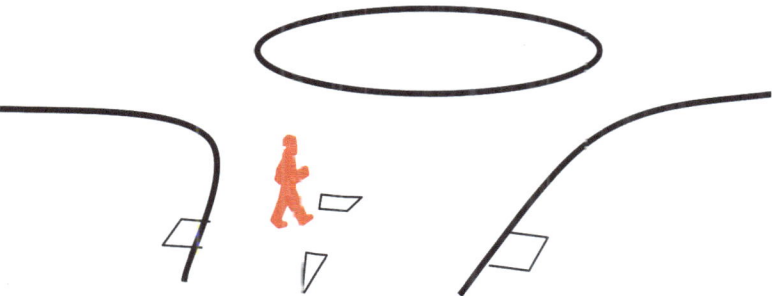

Figure 3.3 Roundabout – a long way to walk

Mini roundabouts, an example of which is shown in Figure 3.4, located at three-way junctions, provide priority to right-turning vehicles at junctions and so inhibit a pedestrian's movement along the major road, as well as across the minor road. This again emphasises the movement of vehicles over pedestrians. Main features of roundabouts and mini roundabouts include:

- higher speed for vehicles due to larger kerb radii at corners and associated intimidation of pedestrians;
- most drivers tend to concentrate on looking to the right when approaching the roundabout in order to give approaching vehicles priority, thereby often not noticing pedestrians crossing from their left;
- excessive distance for crossing pedestrians; and
- pedestrians' desire line disruption.

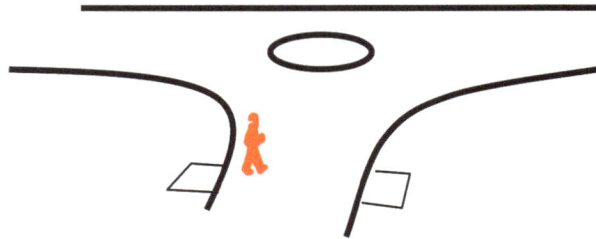

Figure 3.4 Mini roundabout – fast vehicles and often inadequate pedestrian sight distance

A more recent feature of highway facilities is the pedestrian refuge, shown in Figure 3.5. Perhaps inadvertently, its name reveals something of its function. But why should the pedestrian seek 'refuge'? This would seem to imply a need to escape from something. *The Oxford Dictionary* defines the term as "shelter from pursuit or danger". If drivers behave responsibly, why the danger? If a person is crossing the carriageway, the law requires the approaching vehicle to stop or otherwise give priority to the pedestrian.

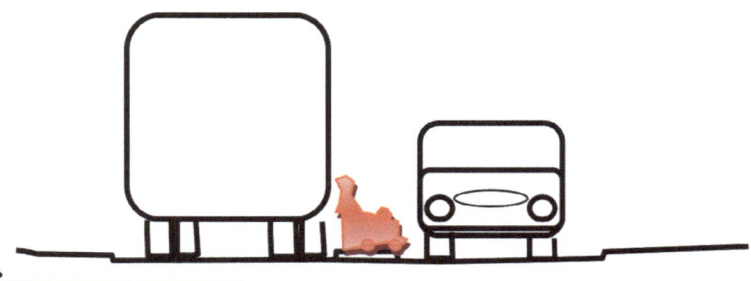

Figure 3.5 Pedestrian refuge in carriageway central reservation

In reality, therefore, the refuge is a convenience for drivers because under the current Highway Code instructions the pedestrian must treat the carriageway as two separate crossings. So approaching vehicles need not stop. Pedestrians have, in effect, to cross twice, so taking longer for the total crossing. In addition, waiting on the refuge is often intimidating. A 20 ton commercial vehicle passing at speed only a foot or so from one's face is not pleasant. Standing at such a refuge with young children is not something that a prudent adult would do. Official recognition of the vulnerability of refuges (but of pedestrians waiting at them) is further evidenced by the provision of flexible vertical markers to enable them to recover from collision with errant vehicles. Is this reassuring to pedestrians?

If the crossing location is such that a refuge needs to be provided, a better solution may be a pedestrian crossing, in recognition of the need for pedestrians' safety and convenience. *Or, perhaps consideration should be given to changing the regulations and the Highway Code so that if a pedestrian has reached a refuge after crossing the first half of the carriageway, approaching vehicles should be required to stop and give the pedestrian priority for the remainder of the crossing.*

Governmental recognition of shortcomings in present design practices is well known; analysis and design approaches and procedures are not based on firm evidence and in some respects are conflicting. As noted in *Manual for Streets* (Department for Transport (DfT) 2007) "Research carried out in the preparation of *Manual for Streets* indicated that many of the criteria routinely applied in street design are based on questionable or outdated practice."

Education of Designers

The subjects of highway and/or traffic engineering are included in most university civil engineering postgraduate degrees in transportation engineering and planning, yet the treatment of pedestrian issues and concerns is limited. The engineering design of road features such as junctions – described in greater detail in Chapter 5 – in order to achieve a design that will avoid collisions between vehicles and pedestrians is an example. Here designers use knowledge of the characteristics of drivers which include: eye movement angle and time; focusing time; reaction time to some event such as seeing a pedestrian start to cross; peripheral vision and head turning angle; and time to view laterally placed features. Considerable research on these items has been completed over many years to establish the relevant values used in design manuals and procedures.

Yet, compared with drivers' characteristics, the only design characteristic of pedestrians who will interact with the driver and vehicles is their walking speed. This ignores, as indicated in Chapter 2, the pedestrian's observation-reaction time before walking, the length of the crossing unit, the time taken to mount the opposite kerb and a safety margin. People who most markedly exhibit these latter requirements include those with small children, older adults, wheelchair and mobility scooter users, and people who diligently and correctly observe the Green Cross Code when crossing.

Thus the higher education of engineers in the essential mathematics and physics design foundations for driver and vehicle behaviour offers few or no applications for the equivalent pedestrian properties. For example, the official *Design Manual for Roads and Bridges (DMRB)* – the technical contents of which are prepared by university-trained engineers – states that in the design of junctions "designers are encouraged to mentally 'drive through' the proposed design…". But no equivalent recommendation is given that designers should 'walk through' the design to ensure its safety for pedestrians. Another instance of lack of attention to pedestrians is that in a well-publicised 150-page book on design of mini roundabouts – one of the most difficult roadway features encountered by pedestrians – they are accorded half a page under the heading 'Miscellaneous'.

Lack of professional involvementt is also evident in basic procedures and documents involved in highway safety – and in the emphasis on motorised traffic. For example, in the Highway Code, lack of clarity in resolving potential conflict between pedestrians and vehicles may result in confusion about accident causes, i.e. involvement of human, environmental or vehicle conditions. The reporting of collisions in the STATS19 system and in collision investigation includes no consideration of pedestrians' abilities, particularly the time taken to look behind them before crossing at junctions – particularly applicable to disabled people.

Unless the investigators are knowledgeable about the detailed physical characteristics and abilities of the pedestrians involved, serious errors can occur in determining the cause of collisions and in structuring solutions. A medical parallel, for example, is that disease outbreaks are often documented through the locations of the victims, their age, the presence of pathogens and exposure to potentially harmful environmental conditions. But unless the medical treatment staff are fully conversant with the detailed biological characteristics of the victims – not merely out-of-date or neglected aspects of their characteristics and condition and often identified in evolving research – a solution to the outbreak is unlikely.

Professional Skills

Concerns have been expressed about the need for improvement in the resources devoted to designing pedestrian facilities. Of note are the areas of professional skills, the guidance on analysis and design of the facilities themselves, and coordination between designers, preparers of the Highway Code and enforcement agencies. The government report *Ending the Scandal of Complacency* (House of Commons, UK Parliament, 2009, para 154) states: "Consistent and adequate long-term funding is required in order to attract and retain the calibre of road safety professional that is required to deliver the road safety strategy."

Several reports and studies have addressed the matter of inadequate skills and training of professionals in the design of pedestrian facilities. For example, the UK Parliament (2002) has addressed many of the perceived problems with the pedestrian environment.

This report addresses issues of national targets, planning, the role of local authorities and specific design approaches. A selection of points particularly relevant to geometric design of pedestrian facilities includes:

- Skills of professionals involved with design for pedestrians are not consistent nationally, and are too often dependent upon selected individuals being responsible for the design process.
- Awareness of the knowledge and skills that are needed for pedestrians appears to be low.
- There is a chronic shortage of professionals, particularly in senior positions, with the appropriate outlook and technical skills.
- There is an unconscious (or conscious) bias of senior officers for car use or at least to concentrate on the problems of traffic congestion and vehicle collisions.
- A chronic shortage of professionals exists, particularly in senior positions, with the appropriate outlook and technical skills.
- Professionals need to pay much more attention to the needs of pedestrians and to the aesthetics of the street. These matters must be addressed in university and other courses and in continued professional development, including the training of officers by local authorities.
- There is a need for consolidated advice which would be used by professionals concerned, including highway engineers, planners and designers. A number of professional institutes and bodies have produced guidance on different aspects of access and mobility, but these need drawing together into a coherent 'Pedestrians' Digest' that allows practitioners to grasp and develop the technical assessment methods that work well.
- There is a need to address the problems of standards being over-rigorously followed, by challenging and justifying existing practices, and encouraging a system of fully trained professionals who provide tailored solutions based upon their professional judgment.

Concerning the adequate funding of improved professional expertise the House of Commons recommendations, paragraph 33 (2009) state:

> Consistent and adequate long-term funding is required in order to attract and retain the calibre of road safety professional that is required to deliver the road safety strategy. (Paragraph 154)

As well as addressing some of the wider issues of designing pedestrian facilities, the report *Paving the Way* (Office of the Deputy Prime Minister (ODPM) and the Commission for Architecture and the Built Environment (CABE) 2002) lists several areas specifically related to geometric design, ranging from the Highway Code to design manuals such as *DMRB*, local transport notes (LTNs) and traffic advisory leaflets (TALs). Selected areas of concern include:

- For priority junctions, lack of emphasis on design for pedestrians and cyclists (*DMRB*, TD 42/95 Part 6).
- For roundabouts, lack of adequate attention to pedestrian facilities (*DMRB*, TD 16/93). Note: this publication has now been updated.
- For signal-controlled junctions and roundabouts, a vehicle flow bias is evident (*DMRB*, TD 50/99).
- Pedestrian crossing design shows an underlying assumption that crossing should be made so as not to inconvenience the driver – this should be revised to emphasise pedestrian traffic flow and comfort.

Highway design guidance and specification for national trunk roads given in *DMRB* includes some specific guidance for urban roads. CABE's (2002:38) comments on this guidance are that:

> … requires greater balance in the geometric and layout presumptions for the design of trunk roads (or other principal routes) in urban areas. Guidance needs to recognise

the greater requirements for pedestrians' access across and along the street and to express clearly whether and how guidance can be used on local roads and what discretion can be used in their interpretation.

Recommendation 2 (CABE 2002:37): Highway Authorities should, under Best Value, establish an audit trail for design decisions affecting the streetscape, to show how design guidance, people's needs and vehicle movements have been accommodated. The aim of this audit trail is twofold:

- To enable local authorities to demonstrate that they have acted 'reasonably' if faced with liability claims. Often the main reason cited for the use of a standard (vehicle priority) solution is that such a solution, however inappropriate to the local context, may offer a line of defence in a court of law.
- To act as a record of aims and objectives about how and why decisions were made, and to show that all users (including disabled people) were considered in the decision-making.

Specific failure in guidance is noted by CABE (2002) in *DMRB*, TD 42/95, Par 6 – Geometric Design of major/minor priority junctions:

- "Assumption that the movement of traffic is the main concern in junction design advantage is that through traffic on the major road is not delayed. No mention is made of advantages for pedestrians and cyclists. Proposed solution: Revise with a more balanced view highlighting advantages for all road users in urban areas where pedestrians and cyclists' needs are higher".
- Also a comment on *DMRB*, TD 16/93: "Where the conflict between pedestrians and vehicles at roundabouts is mentioned pedestrian facilities are promoted away from the junction point, and a guardrail is required to prevent 'indiscriminate' crossing".

Regarding visibility splays the Institution of Civil Engineers' (2000) *Designing Streets for People* report states: "Visibility splays greatly influence the street scene. Guidance on dimensions for visibility splays is given in 'Places, Streets and Movements' but the rationale behind the figures is not. Therefore, there is no basis for a professional to understand, interpret or question the guidance. However, if the scientific justification behind the figures were published, the guidance could be understood and applied to local circumstances."

Vocational and Further Education

Relatively few people currently working on road safety have formal or comprehensive training in this specific field, according to *Road Safety Good Practice Guide: Road Safety Qualifications* (DfT, Section 2.34, undated). The guide further states: "However, many may have been trained in associated disciplines, such as civil engineering, teaching or traffic management. In general, safety personnel have gained their valuable knowledge through observation and on-the-job experience. Some have also attended seminars or been on short training courses, for example in the use of specialised software."

Other safety training available includes: a two-week Royal Society for the Prevention of Accidents (RoSPA) road safety engineering course; a one-week course for road safety officers; road safety courses for local authority staff; miscellaneous road safety audit courses; other miscellaneous road safety courses; and miscellaneous software training workshops. This list is not comprehensive and several other courses are available within the UK.

Examination of the content of most of these courses does not indicate the depth of knowledge, either theoretical or practical, which adequately addresses pedestrian needs to the extent that they are applicable to detailed design of safe and convenient pedestrian facilities for all road users.

Particularly lacking in the educational background of engineers and planners are the access and mobility needs of disabled people – all of them ambulatory road users, of whom all are at some time pedestrians. A review of civil, highway and traffic engineering curricula at a selection of twelve British universities revealed that only one included design of facilities for disabled pedestrians on the syllabus. This consisted of one two-hour presentation of key issues addressing legislation, categories of disability, physical abilities of disabled people and official guidelines on street and public transport facilities.

Pedestrian Facilities as a Consumer Product

Most products available to the public, from the pull-tabs on sardine cans to air bags in cars, are designed and constructed to ensure operation without injuring their users. The design features of these products often require detailed, informed, technical knowledge in order to produce a safe, efficient product. If they were not safe they would quickly lose buyers, and public pressure for governmental regulation would mandate acceptable safety levels. Recalls of cars because of safety deficiencies are well documented.

How would we consider footways, crossings, barriers, signs and other features affecting pedestrians as a consumer product, i.e. something we had bought (we have, through our taxes) and expected to be safe and convenient to use? How would it compare with other products that we use daily? Would its designers want to ensure a successful product that sold well and was not recalled because of dangerous features? In other words, would its designers be judged lacking if this 'product' did not generate more safe and convenient walking trips? While we may not view pedestrian facilities in quite the same light, perhaps concerns as if it were a product would encourage improved performance – especially greater safety – for its users. We can but hope.

★

> The bias in the emphasis on provision of features related to motor vehicles in the highway and street system is, perhaps, understandable from the point of view of those responsible for design and implementation. Most designers are car owners and users, and their approach is influenced by the overwhelming societal culture of the car and its employment in day-to-day activities. Unfortunately, such biases are reflected in the lack of education and training of design professionals, as indicated by concerned groups and institutions. *Emphasis on pedestrian infrastructure design at undergraduate and/or, preferably, master's level, needs a curriculum at least equivalent to that provided for drivers and vehicle-based highway design – especially as regards safety matters.* Recognition of how current biases can affect the safety and convenience of pedestrians can lead to improvements – many of which are described in the relevant chapters – but concerted action both in education and outlook in terms of pedestrians' safety and convenience will be needed.

References

Department for Transport (2007) *Manual for Streets*. Thomas Telford, London.

Department for Transport (Undated) *Road Safety Good Practice Guide, Road Safety Qualifications,* Section 2.34, U-GOV website.

House of Commons Transport Committee (2009) *Ending the Scandal of Complacency: Road Safety Beyond 2010.* Second Special Report of Session 2008-09, p.3. London.

Office of the Deputy Prime Minister and the Commission for Architecture and the Built Environment (2002) *Paving the Way*. Thomas Telford, London.

Schoon, J.G. and Hounsell, N.B. (2006) *Access and mobility design policy for disabled pedestrians at road crossings: exploration of issues.* Transportation Research Record, Journal of the Transportation Research Board. 1956, 76-85. (doi:10.3141/1956-10)

UK Government (2004) Section 16 of the Traffic Management Act 2004.

UK Parliament (2002) Select Committee on Environment, Transport and Regional Affairs. Eleventh Report, *Walking in Towns and Cities*. London.

CHAPTER 4

FORENSIC ANALYSIS

Are we learning?

Have you ever been injured by an exploding bottle of lemonade? Probably not – but not for lack of care and attention. Most consumer products and services have benefited from rigorous analysis to eliminate accidents and malfunctions. Often, such investigation is legally mandated not only to determine liability in the event of a mishap but to provide essential feedback to design and operations. Examples include the airlines' requirement for investigating crash or other dangerous events – and resulting directives for remedies. Reported road collisions and the resulting investigations can similarly help to identify deficiencies and guide improvements. But the methods for getting and transferring useful information to achieve them are often fragmented and unclear. As a result, lack of suitable data and analysis methods hinder the responsive design and operation of junctions, crossings and other facilities needed for pedestrian safety. Here we review key current forensic methods and how they might improve pedestrian safety.

★

Need for and Role of Forensic Analysis

The need for forensic analysis of road accidents is well understood. Julie Townsend, Deputy Chief Executive at Brake, the road safety charity, commented to the Association of Chief Police Officers (ACPO 2012), "… we learn from collisions to prevent further tragedies; police work liaising with victims and investigating crashes is fundamental to this." Further, the *Road Death Investigation Manual* (ACPO 2007) addresses wider issues and states that:

The primary function of forensic examination is to identify and secure evidence. It also provides the roads policing senior investigating officer (RPSIO) with an understanding of what happened at the scene, even when this is not of direct evidential value. For these reasons the RPSIO should think about the application of forensic investigation techniques in their widest sense and not from a purely evidential perspective.

As there are continual advancements in forensic investigation techniques, RPSIOs may have difficulty in keeping abreast of changes in this field. Some familiarity with the potential applications of forensic investigation techniques and forensic science will, however, be of significant help. RPSIOs should endeavour to maintain their professional knowledge in these areas but do not need scientific expertise. This specific knowledge is available from, for example, collision investigators and scientific advisers. It is the role of the RPSIO to harness such expertise to further an investigation.

Two important ways to improve the highway system to reduce the number of accidents are in use: forensic analysis of individual events, and recording of individual accident circumstances which can be analysed statistically at national or other levels, typically done using the STATS19 system (DfT 2013) – a system which records frequency and causes of accidents throughout the UK.

Benefits of Forensic Analysis

Collisions between pedestrians and vehicles must be analysed to apportion responsibility for causing and/or contributing to a collision (with the associated insurance and legal implications) and to obtain data which can guide improvements to:

- infrastructure, such as geometric layout affecting sight lines;
- operational practices such as traffic signal design and operation;
- location of signs and other features controlling the interaction between pedestrians and vehicles; and,
- detailed structural features of infrastructure, such as skid resistance of the pavement and surface roughness of the footway.

History

As reported by Field (2001), road traffic accident reconstruction began in the USA in the early 1960s. Training of police began in the UK in 1970 based on material developed by the Metropolitan Police forensic science branch. Currently, police officers who have successfully undertaken a course and obtained a certificate in forensic road accident reconstruction through the City and Guilds (C & G) of London Institute are qualified to provide expert testimony in court on the events associated with a collision. Initially, while undertaking the C & G course, an officer undergoes supervised work training under a senior collision investigator. 'Basic' and 'Standard' levels of qualification are obtained and then, upon achievement of 'Advanced' status, and having obtained the C & G qualification, the officer can then cite his or her qualifications in reports or statements.

The C & G qualification is granted only to people employed by police authorities. Otherwise people wishing to obtain the relevant qualifications may undertake the University Certificate in Continuing Professional Development in Forensic Road Collision Investigation, usually by distance learning.

Initially, accident scene investigation should include human, vehicle and environmental factors which include, but are not confined to:

Human Factors

- Alcohol and/or drugs
- Vehicle occupant restraint use – were restraints correctly worn?
- Fatigue
- Bad or injudicious driving
- Distraction of the driver, road user, pedestrian, e.g. through use of a mobile phone
- Health and eyesight issues
- Training and competence of the driver or road user
- Other road user or pedestrian movements

Vehicle Factors

- Roadworthiness and general condition
- Suitability of vehicle for use or location, e.g. moped on a motorway
- Potential design fault, e.g. an inbuilt blind spot

Environmental Factors

- Road condition, e.g. condition of the road surface
- Road geometry, e.g. curvature and grade
- Roadside protection, e.g. purpose and condition of the central reservation barriers
- Signage, lighting, automatic traffic signals
- Weather conditions at the time of the collision

Research and Analysis

The causes and characteristics of road accidents are done internationally by academic investigators and the results are published in a wide variety of academic and professional journals. *There is, however, no mandatory updating of skills or expertise among practising police accident investigators.*

Reportedly (Field 2001) in a study selected eight technical papers published between 1995 and 2003 which addressed various aspects of road accident reconstruction methods. Topics of the papers included data on vehicle speed, road friction, analysis of pedestrian collision types, calculation of impact speed, theoretical vs empirically derived solutions for vehicle/pedestrian collision and characteristics of pedestrian trajectory when struck by a vehicle. All of these matters affect the accuracy of reconstruction methods and procedures. Police responses to the papers were categorised as: read, used, no comment, not heard of.

The results of the study make disturbing reading; *a key finding is that less than 2% of the respondents had even heard of seven of the papers and that although 52% had heard of the remaining paper, only 3% had read it.* Clearly, reliance on the results of police forensic analysis may need some review.

A prerequisite to much of the accident analysis is a mathematically based understanding of the static and dynamic characteristics of the vehicle, driver and pedestrian, and environmental features such as road geometry, lighting and skid resistance. Of key importance to achieving the desired result is the need for a recognised, mandatory procedure involving relevant government legislation, ministerial authority, implementing agency involvement and enforcement.

Organisations that regularly use Department for Transport's (DfT's) road safety data include Transport Research Laboratory (TRL); Transport Safety Research Centre, Loughborough University; Centre for Transport Studies, University College London; the Parliamentary Advisory Council on Transport Safety (PACTS); and the Royal Society for the Prevention of Accidents (RoSPA). All of these organisations, as well as other mainly academic institutions, contribute to advances in, and greater knowledge of, the characteristics of collisions, yet there is no recognised method of reviewing and including useful results into practice.

Reporting

Reporting of road accidents on the public highway which involve human injury or death in Great Britain is done by police officers onto a STATS19 form – the basic means of documenting details of the collision. The first statistics were collected in 1979 and have been made available annually since then. DfT has overall responsibility for the design and collection system of the STATS19 data. The Standing Committee on Road Accident Statistics (SCRAS) is the body set up to oversee the STATS19 process.

The STATS19 form assembles a wide variety of information about the accident (such as time, date, location, road conditions, vehicles and casualties) and contributory factors to the accident as interpreted by the police. The form is completed at either the scene of the accident, or when the accident is reported to the police. However, it is not a complete record of all injuries, since some accidents (mostly minor ones) may not come to the attention of the police, and hospitals may have different information.

National road accident statistics inform public debate and provide the basis for determining and monitoring targeted road safety policies – a process that requires consistent and accurate data recording of casualties. National and local government and local police forces work closely to achieve a common reporting standard. The results of the data collection are used for research and for guidance in improving safety.

Local authorities use road accident data extensively – engineers for establishing priority sites for remedial measures and road safety officers for national and local educational programmes and training. Collected data is also used by a range of establishments for academic and governmental research into road safety measures.

Augmenting the STATS19 process, the STATS20 document provides instructions to police officers to enable completion of the STATS19 form, and the STATS21 document (not generally available to the public) covers the validity checks, error procedures and submission of the STATS19 data.

The data sources do not contain items that might be disclosive, such as drivers' and casualties' postcodes, breath test information and contributory factors towards an accident. Data from the two different sources cannot be linked due to differences in the record identifier codes.

Data quality may be affected by police definitions of serious injury covering casualties admitted to hospital, as well as those with specific types of injury (for example, fractures or severe cuts). This means that in theory all patients in hospital emergency services (HES) admitted following a road traffic accident should also appear as seriously injured casualties in the police report. But in practice not all road casualties are reported to the police. Also, apparently in some cases casualties that meet the definition of a serious injury are only recorded by the police as slight. However, comparisons with death registration statistics show that very few, if any, road accident fatalities are not reported to the police.

The cause of reported road accidents is not collected on the STATS19 form. However, information on factors which, in the opinion of the police officer who attended the scene of a reported road accident, may have contributed to the accident is collected, but would only be available under special licence from DfT.

Investigation of Accidents Involving Pedestrians

Imperfect knowledge and application of a pedestrian's crossing actions may result in the incorrect conclusions of a particular forensic analysis. Walking time across a carriageway, although the most common pedestrian activity when a collision occurs, is typically calculated using only walking speed expressed as an average value of the pedestrian crossing the carriageway multiplied by the distance walked. As indicated in Chapter 2, specific items not included in current pedestrian trajectory and timing are a pedestrian's initial observation-reaction time (including the time for the crossing unit to cross the footway to the kerb), the length of the crossing unit and a safety margin when the unit reaches the opposite kerb.

An example of incorrect conclusions using conventional methods about a pedestrian collision could be where a pedestrian crosses at a marked crossing (such as a dropped kerb on the minor arm of a priority junction) which does not have adequate pedestrian sight distance to approaching vehicles, as shown in Figure 4.1(a) where:

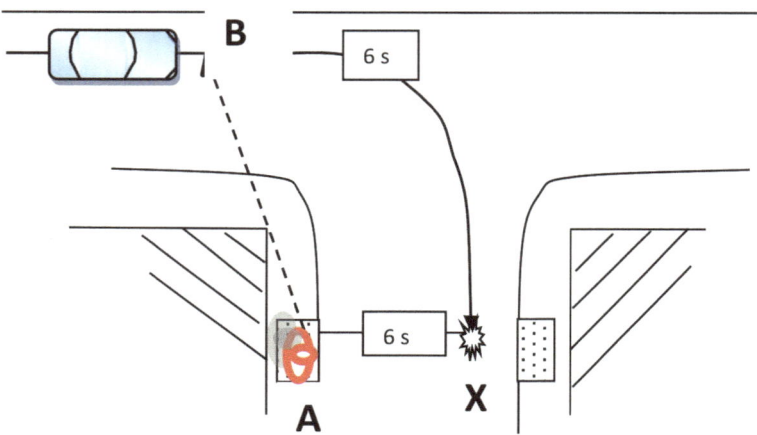

Figure 4.1(a) Trajectories with conventional pedestrian crossing time estimation

- A is the point at which the pedestrian would start to cross.
- B is the point immediately to the left of which the pedestrian could not see the vehicle (shaded) approaching.
- X is the point at which the pedestrian and vehicle would collide.
- AB is the pedestrian's available sight line to point B.
- The conventional way to estimate the pedestrian's time from

the kerb to the collision point would be to divide the distance AX (measured on site) by only the walking speed, resulting in a time of, say 5 seconds.

The pedestrian at A, after looking per the Green Cross Code starts to walk although unable to see the approaching vehicle on the main road due to the obstruction of the corner when viewed (as shown by the broken line) from the designated crossing point. The driver, distracted or otherwise unaware, takes no avoiding action and collides with the pedestrian at X.

If in the accident reporting and reconstruction the estimated speed of the vehicle were to place the vehicle just outside the pedestrian's range of vision (just to the left of point B) when he started to walk then the pedestrian's 'contributory factors' to the collision with the STATS 19 reference numbers could be incorrectly listed as:

- *802 Failure to look properly*
- *803 Failed to judge vehicle's path or speed*
- *808 Careless, reckless or in a hurry*

… even though the pedestrian could not see the approaching vehicle before he or she walked.

But it actually would have *taken the pedestrian 9 sec to reach point X instead of 6 sec (because of having to observe, react and move from the kerb before starting to walk)* and in order to avoid collision he or she would have had to see the vehicle approaching at point C, which was impossible due to the position of the drop kerb and the obstruction, as shown in Figure 4.1(b).

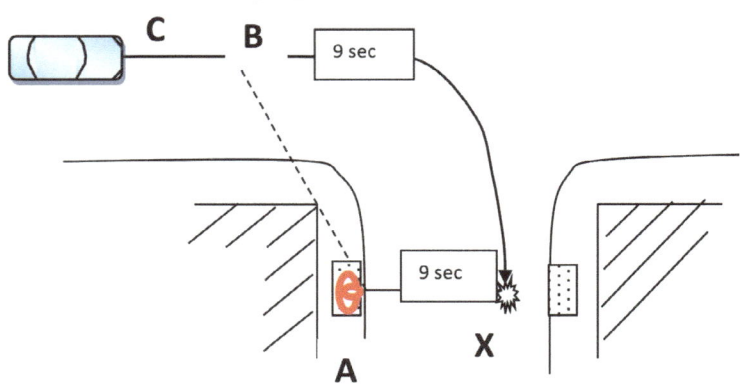

Figure 4.1(b) Trajectories with full pedestrian crossing time requirement time estimation

Hence, the STATS19 system, combined with the incorrect knowledge about the pedestrian's abilities, would have failed in its role of providing a basis for indicating infrastructure design flaws because the collision would have been incorrectly attributed to one or more of the above listed 'contributory factors' on the pedestrian's part. Therefore, indications of needed infrastructure improvements (i.e. redesign of pedestrian crossing locations and/or removal of pedestrian sight line obstruction, or reduction in speed limit) would not be evident. Also, the pedestrian would be considered to be at least partly at fault in causing the collision.

Crucially also, based on the available listing of contributory factors on the STATS19 form, there is no available category for indicating that the pedestrian had insufficient sight distance for deciding to start to cross. Whereas drivers and riders may warrant a contributory factor on the STATS19 form of "Vision affected by", i.e:

> 703 Road Layout (e.g. bend, winding road, hill crest). Only use this code where driver's/rider's vision was affected by the road layout (e.g. failing to see pedestrian crossing at bend, or a vehicle overtaking near crest of hill).

... there is no equivalent contributory factor that identifies problems which pedestrians may have with road layout, and which contribute to their injury and death.

Deficiencies related to a collision can be categorised as user error, vehicle and/or highway defect (including signage and other appurtenances of the latter). Combining these with pre-crash, crash and post-crash conditions enables a useful matrix for analysis. Table 4.1 shows a tabular summary of the collision described above and its outcome under the assumption that the pedestrian's walking speed alone was the basis for the collision reconstruction, resulting in a walking time of 6 sec. Contrast this with Table 4.2 showing the equivalent format but under the assumption that the pedestrian took 9 sec to reach the collision point.

TIME SCALE	HUMAN		VEHICLE	ENVIRONMENT
	Pedestrian	Driver[1]		
Pre-crash	No fault	Distracted	None	No inadequacies
Crash	Partially at fault	Distracted	None	No inadequacies

(1) Driver distraction during period needed for avoidance action.

Table 4.1 Collision reconstruction outcome using only pedestrian's average walking speed

TIME SCALE	HUMAN		VEHICLE	ENVIRONMENT
	Pedestrian	Driver[1]		
Pre-crash	No fault	Distracted	None	Inadequate sight line to approaching vehicles
Crash	No fault	Disracted	None	

(1) Driver distraction during period needed for avoidance action.

Table 4.2 Collision reconstruction outcome using pedestrian's observation-reaction time and unit length in addition to average walking speed

Potential Liability Issues

Given the numerical basis for the outcome with the variables described, it is evident that a factual, calculable risk of a collision exists between the pedestrian and the vehicle, assuming that the crossing location is a part of a pedestrian's route for his or her necessary activities. In parallel terms of product liability, if a product were to pose the risk of injury when a consumer wished to use it in the approved fashion (similar to a pedestrian using the Green Cross Code before crossing) then the maker of the product could be considered responsible for the consumer's injury. The implications of this for the design of many junctions and other locations where pedestrians have insufficient sight distance are unclear, and research is urgently needed to clarify the issues and establish satisfactory design guidance.

It must also be noted that a driver, even although driving carefully, may fail to see the pedestrian and/or take avoiding action for a number of reasons beyond his or her control. External environmental factors and the phenomenon of 'looked but did not see' (Brown 2006) often may be the sole or contributory cause of the collision. However, about 44% of all accidents are identified by the term 'failed to look properly' plus a number of other reasons including speeding and excessive alcohol use.

Future Directions for Forensic Analysis

From the point of view of future pedestrian safety the current reconstruction of pedestrian actions would not contribute to improved design practice because although the mathematical method was itself correct (i.e. the estimation of distances travelled by the vehicle) *the assumptions about the pedestrian's actions did not include the pedestrian's observation-reaction time, or length of the walking unit*. Most forensic accident reconstruction methods emphasise pedestrian 'throw' distance as a means of calculating vehicle speed, if not otherwise known. Although this is useful in investigating the cause of the final collision it would not necessarily assist in identifying shortcomings in the layout and dimensions of the junction or other location where pedestrian sight distance is essential to the pedestrian crossing safely.

Summarising several key features of STATS19 where only driver/rider actions can be recorded: Codes 702, 703 and 704 each relate to driver/rider vision as affected by vegetation, road layout and buildings and related features respectively, and are to be identified. There is no provision for recording that a pedestrian's vision was affected by any of these items. Therefore, adequate information about key features of the collision which could lead to improved facilities design and operations may well be missed.

Improving safety by implementing new designs begins with on-site review and measurement of individual accidents in a standardised fashion, recorded in STATS19 and analysed over extended periods. The results are converted to statistically relevant features which can contribute to adding new, or modifying existing, design guidance. The process can be shown diagrammatically in Figure 4.2, and summarised as follows:

> **Items 1 and 2.** Accidents as they occur in the road network have specific features of the collision which, if adequately recorded, can be analysed to improve pedestrian safety. Deficiencies in identifying pedestrian categories exist, including the recording of pedestrians in wheelchairs and those accompanied by guide dogs or otherwise assisted.
>
> **Item 3**. The details of the specific accident are recorded and reconstruction conducted by police if required for prosecution or related purposes. Potential issues include:

- The accident features to be recorded must include the details of the collision and environment which contribute to the accident. An example omission affecting pedestrian accidents is that there is no item on the STATS19 form to record, under 'contributory factors', inadequate visibility for pedestrians where such visibility distance is needed to permit them to see approaching vehicles in time to cross safely. This matter is related to 'intervisibility' as used in design procedures in the *Design Manual for Roads and Bridges (DMRB)*, where the concept does not recognise that pedestrians require a greater time to physically react to an approaching vehicle than the driver requires when reacting to a crossing pedestrian. See also Chapter 5.

- Pedestrian crossing behaviour and characteristics need to be correctly understood and quantified in order to calculate relative pedestrian and vehicle times and distances to the collision point. The STATS19 form has no provision for recording pedestrians' observation-reaction times, length of crossing unit (particularly important concerning disabled pedestrians, wheelchair movement or people with prams and small children) and time to cross the footway prior to entering the carriageway. See also Chapter 2.

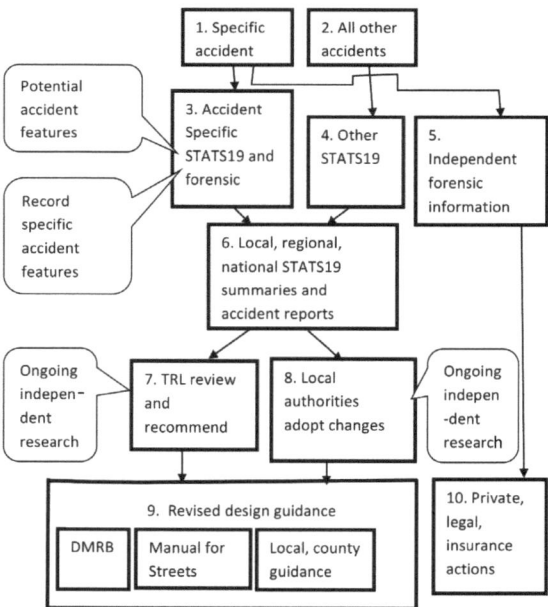

Figure 4.2 Road design improvement process from accident records to design manuals – an outline

Item 4. Other STATS19 reports are completed – with the same issues as in Item 3, above.

Item 5. Often, where action is to be taken for insurance or legal reasons, a forensic analysis may be undertaken by an independent firm or consultant for use by the affected parties. This analysis often relies at least partly on the police STATS19 report and related documents.

Item 6. STATS19 reports are made available to interested parties.

Item 7. TRL, as contractor to DfT, researches selected issues in order to provide evidence for changes in design guidance in *DMRB* and *MfS*, and to inform local and county authorities of new guidance. Issues affecting improvements include:

- TRL is a contractor to DfT. Therefore, unless DfT identifies relevant areas of problems it cannot contract with research organisations such as TRL to investigate specific issues, such as those mentioned in Item 3, above.
- Researchers at TRL must be aware of relevant research in order to adequately contribute to design improvements.

Item 8. Local authorities, in viewing the research results of TRL, are free to adopt the guidance or not. A potential issue is whether the authority chooses to do so, resulting in uneven application of design approaches throughout the UK.

Item 9. Changes of guidance are, in time, incorporated into *DMRB* and *Manual for Streets* and into local and county guidance documents. The time frame for doing this does not seem to be regular, and needed changes may be delayed beyond the time when evidence suggests they would be beneficial.

Item 10. Individual forensic analyses are used as appropriate for legal and/or insurance purposes. Where persistent and clear repetition of accident causes becomes apparent, it is possible that the remedial measures may be transmitted to DfT and to local and county authorities as a basis for changes in design guidance.

Governmental Recognition

Shortcomings in the accident reporting and forensic analysis system are shown in the House of Commons Transport Committee report (2009) where the specific items related to investigative analysis are described as follows:

Item 21. It is anomalous that the vast majority of work-related deaths are not examined by the Health and Safety Executive, purely because they occur on the roads. The Government should review the role of the Health and Safety Executive with regard to road safety to ensure that it fulfils its unique role in the strategy beyond 2010.

Item 34. The approach taken to investigating accidents differs sharply across the transport modes and there is insufficient cross-over between road and the other modes. The systems approach that is routine in marine, rail and aviation accident investigation and prevention is much less apparent in road safety. The Government should facilitate greater exchange of personnel, ideas and learning across the modes.

Item 35. A road accident investigation branch should be formed, to parallel those for aviation, marine and rail. Its purpose would be to draw together lessons from the fatal accident investigations undertaken by police and other sources. (Paragraph 157)

Regarding the STATS19 system of recording road traffic accidents, it is further recommended that an independent review be made in order to establish its strengths and weaknesses, when considering the recommendations above for a British road safety survey. The review should also examine possible simplification, promotion of greater consistency, and routine linking of police and hospital data.

Discouraging Walking

It will be evident from the foregoing that unless adequate sight distance exists for pedestrians to see approaching vehicles their attempts at crossing can only be made on the assumption that a driver will see them in time to avoid a collision. Thus, the pedestrian cannot be in control of his or her own safety, and therefore he or she will be discouraged from walking, with the resulting health, wellbeing and economic implications. This is particularly true for people who may have to cross slowly due to some encumbrance of disability. Lack of information on the numbers of people so affected is limited, but if the 12% of disabled people in Britain are affected in this way, more than 8 million people either cannot, or are discouraged from, walking.

Independent Organisation Interests

As well as government agencies many independent organisations are concerned with effective investigation of road casualties. We conclude with one example (Roadpeace 2016), which in its listing embodies some of the concerns with current approaches and the need for improvement:

What RoadPeace wants (RoadPeace2016)
More effective investigations, with:

- Nationally agreed standards of good practice
- Trained collision investigators with national accreditation

- Proper quality assurance, ensuring processes are monitored and maintained
- Risk reduced through better analysis and design of countermeasures tackling danger at source
- Improvements in injury investigation as well as road death and life changing collision investigation.

★

> The many organisations and fragmented responsibilities, combined with incomplete review of relevant research by official and private interests, has resulted in an inefficient transfer of forensically derived information into practical design measures to improve pedestrian safety. The examples given of the ways in which pedestrians' actions can be misinterpreted through use of the current STATS19 system of recording and/or not being recorded at all can lead to gross errors in understanding the causes of collisions and, therefore, ways to reduce them. Beyond the current framework, potential avenues of improvement clearly need to be explored. These would include a comprehensive systems approach, recognition of the detailed capabilities of pedestrians described earlier, possible implementation of an independent accident investigation branch similar to air and marine interests, more inclusive consideration of pedestrian issues in STATS19, and the possibility of involving the Health and Safety Executive in collision investigation. Furthermore, a more effective system needs to have a complete review at ministerial level as a basis for legislating measurable improvements in pedestrian safety.

References

Association of Chief Police Officers (2007) *Police Road Death Investigation Manual,* p. 65. London.

Brown, I. (2006) Road Safety Research Report No 60 Transport Research Laboratory. Theme 2: *Driver and Rider Behaviour Crowthorne*. DfT website www.dft.gov.uk.

Association of Chief Police Officers (2012) Media Centre – Internet: *Public Invited to Contribute to Police Road Death Investigation Policy,* 8 August 2012, London.

Department for Transport (2013) *Road Accidents and Safety Statistics Guidance. STATS19 Road Accident Injury Statistics Report Form*. London.

Field, J. (2001) *Getting it Right*. West Midlands Police, Birmingham, UK.

House of Commons Transport Committee (2009) *Ending the Scandal of Complacency: Road Safety Beyond 2010. Second Special Report of Session 2008–09*, p.3. London.

RoadPeace. Website accessed February 2016.

Further reading

Collision investigation is a complex and continually evolving science, well beyond the points discussed in this chapter. Several books which readers may find helpful in becoming more familiar with the issues, mainly from a driver's point of view, are listed below:

Evans, L., (2004) *Traffic Safety*. www.Science Serving Society.com or Amazon.

Groeger, J.A. (2000). *Understanding Driving: applying cognitive psychology to a complex everyday task*. Psychology Press, Hove.

Hole, G.J. (2007) *The Psychology of Driving*. Earlbaum Associates Hove.

Olson, P.L. and Farber, E. (2003) *Forensic Aspect s of Driver Perception and Response (Second Edition)*. Lawyrers and Judges Publishing Co. Tucson. Arizona.

CHAPTER 5

JUNCTIONS AND OTHER CROSSINGS

Survival of the fleetest?

You will need to look in at least four different directions within a few seconds before safely walking across even one arm of a simple three-way junction. Here, interaction is between pedestrians and vehicles which often approach together and, suddenly, from several directions. Obstructed sight lines, and limited space for pedestrians to stand and/or manoeuvre before crossing add to the danger – evidenced by the many accidents at these places. Crossings at straight sections of road and near bends where pedestrian traffic occurs exhibit many of the features of junctions, especially with respect to the interaction of visibility, vehicle speeds and pedestrians' abilities. Current crossing designs present many problems for drivers and pedestrians. Now we look at some of their features and potential ways to make them safer.

★

The Basic Priority Junction

Although stating the obvious, a junction of two or more roads enables traffic, including pedestrian traffic, to change direction in order to link origins and destinations. A major feature of junction design is to enable these changes in direction to be made efficiently and safely. As with other features of transport the definition of 'efficient' often ignores the matter of equity and, too often, pedestrians rank below vehicles. Unfortunately, the complexity of only one junction or a bend in the road can render a walking route inadvisable, difficult or, for some people, impossible and so discourage walking in general.

Consider the most simple of junctions, the 'T' or 'priority junction' as it is called in technical terms, typical examples of which are shown in the diagrammatic sketches of Figure 5.1, and where no traffic signals are present – by far the most common type of junction. This junction has a major road of two or more lanes and a minor road of two lanes. The main road is typically a radial trunk road in suburbs or nearer the town centre, where a minor road joins it.

Common needs of pedestrians are to walk to and then along the footways of major roads to visit suburban shops or to walk to and from the town centre. These areas are often not the focus of intense pedestrian activity such as in town centres with many traffic signals, but nevertheless may include as many as twenty crossings on such a trip. Here, pedestrians face a variety of signs, footway shapes and kerb alignments. Ramps assist people in wheelchairs, scooters and pedestrians with prams. They then have to look for approaching vehicles and decide on the safest way to cross: directly across, at the end of a radius, set in from the major road, or possibly a combination of these.

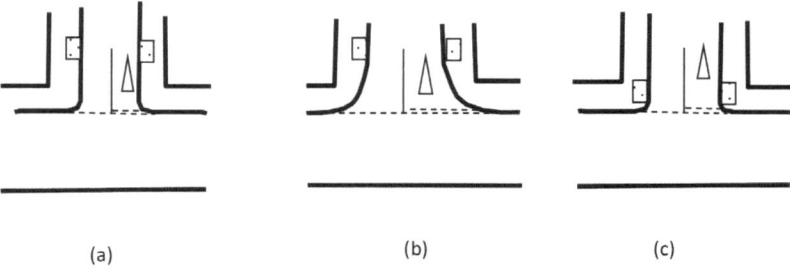

(a)   (b)   (c)

Figures 5.1(a), (b) and (c) Examples of crossing locations for pedestrians on minor arm of junction – diagrammatic

But when the crossing points are set back from the kerbline of the major road, as shown in Figures 5.1(a) and (b), the general rule of vehicular and pedestrian traffic proceeding straight along the major road having priority (Highway Code Rule 170), as in Figure 1(c), is negated for pedestrians and they must cross the minor road where vehicles turn faster and where sight lines to approaching vehicles are shorter.

Vehicular traffic travelling straight on the major road takes priority over turning traffic. The basis for this is that the higher volumes of traffic are moving in a straight direction, and are usually travelling faster than turning traffic. It follows, therefore, that this straight ahead traffic takes priority over the turning traffic. In Britain, cars, trucks, horses, bicycles, motorbikes all have this priority at a junction. *But pedestrians only have this priority if they put themselves in danger by venturing from the kerb onto the carriageway of the minor arm in order to attain their legal priority over any turning vehicle.* Other difficulties from turning vehicles are present, as discussed in more detail in Chapter 6 on the Highway Code. In addition, pedestrians are often required to divert from, and add distance to, their route, as shown in Figure 5.2. Also, because the minor road may also be on a gradient from the junction, this can cause greater difficulties for disabled people, especially those in wheelchairs or using other mobility aids, or for people accompanied by small children.

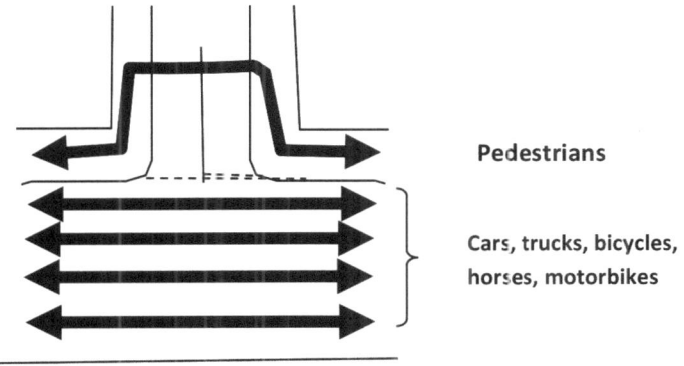

Figure 5.2 Frequent divergent route for pedestrians at junctions compared with other modes

Conventional design justification for not providing direct crossing for pedestrians includes the recommendation that vehicles turning from the major arms should not be delayed as this will tend to reduce the capacity of the major road. Also, it is considered that drivers are likely to collide with the vehicle in front which has to slow down to allow the pedestrians to cross the minor road entrance. Further, it has been stated that the pedestrian's position enables drivers turning to better see pedestrians waiting to cross or crossing (not that pedestrians can better see approaching vehicles). This diminishes the priority that pedestrians have for continuing across the minor arm parallel with the major traffic flows. It also tends to negate the general rule that traffic (including pedestrians and cyclists) moving straight ahead has priority over turning traffic.

Conflict Characteristics

According to the Highway Code, pedestrians have priority when crossing an arm into which a vehicle is turning (Rule 170), as shown in Figures 5.3, 5.4 and 5.5. These pedestrian movements include those where the pedestrian is crossing the major road arms and a vehicle is turning into the major road from the minor road. However, this pedestrian priority is not emphasised or illustrated graphically, as described in Chapter 6. In addition, the Code states (for drivers): "The approach to a junction may have a 'Give Way' sign or a triangle marked on the road. You **MUST** give way to traffic on the main road when emerging from a junction with broken white lines across the road." Since pedestrians are 'traffic' (Legislation UK gov.com, Traffic Management Act, Section 31, 2004), this rule applies to pedestrians also, but drivers may not equate 'main road' with the footway parallel with the main road.

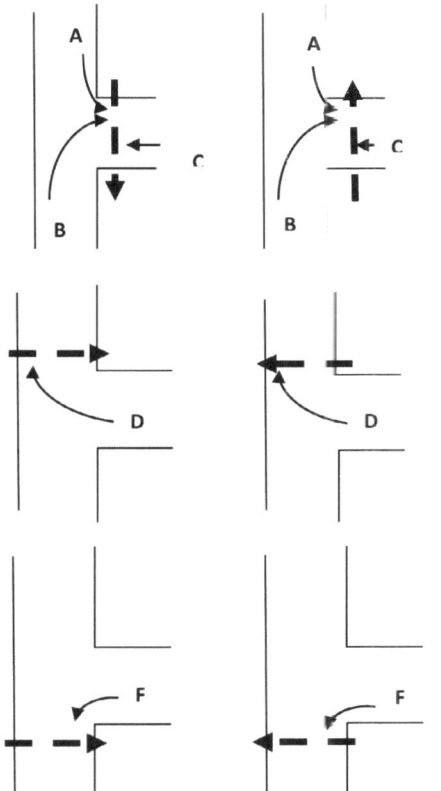

Figure 5.3 Pedestrian/vehicle conflicts: pedestrian crossing minor arm of junction conflicts with left- and right-turning vehicles A and B from major arm and straight ahead vehicle C on minor arm.

Figure 5.4 Pedestrian/vehicle conflicts: pedestrian crossing major arm of junction conflicts with right-turning vehicle D from minor arm.

Figure 5.5 Pedestrian/vehicle conflicts: pedestrian crossing major arm of junction conflicts with left-turning vehicle F from minor arm.

In accordance with the abilities and actions of pedestrians wishing to cross (outlined in Chapter 2), the movement of approaching vehicles and the geometric layout and dimensions of the crossing must be considered in the junction's design. An example is the case of a pedestrian wishing to cross the minor arm of a junction, as shown in the sketch of Figure 5.6. The pedestrian must look and focus in at least four directions as part of the necessary observation before starting to cross. It is obvious from this that a pedestrian will have periods of time when 'blind' to movements in a different direction in which he or she is looking, because it takes a finite amount of time to turn one's head and shoulders and to focus on approaching vehicles. The relevance of this situation is reflected to some extent in a court judgement (Berrymans Lace Mawer 2008) where "… a pedestrian was rarely a danger to anyone else and that he had to look to both sides as well as forwards. A motorist did not have to look sideways and if he failed to keep a look out the consequences could be disastrous. It was quite possible, therefore, for a motorist to be much more to blame than the pedestrian."

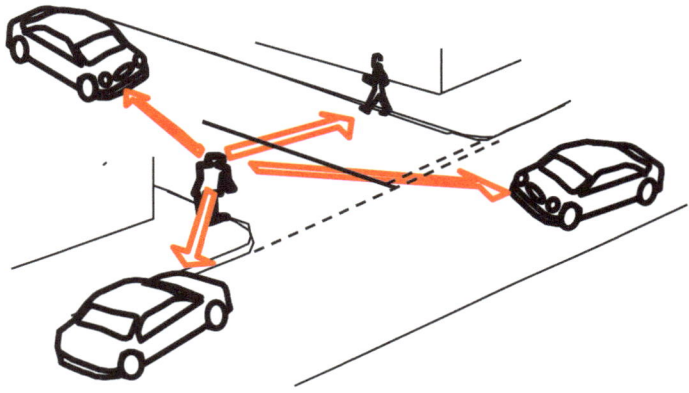

Figure 5.6 Directions in which pedestrians must look and focus before starting to cross in accordance with the Green Cross Code

These directions of looking are embedded in the rules for crossing based on the *Green Cross Code and the Highway Code*, i.e. looking all around, and so involving a scanning and focusing sweep of nearly 260 degrees, which for a pedestrian about to cross is as shown in the diagram of Figure 5.7. As described in the chapter on pedestrian characteristics, focusing is an often unrecognised and unappreciated aspect of the pedestrian's observation process. In order to focus on a vehicle approaching and to judge its speed accurately (not merely see it) – and hence decide if it is safe to cross – takes significant time. Two seconds to focus may seem long but at 20 mph a vehicle travels 60 ft (18 m), and the 'car that came from nowhere' has too often proved lethal.

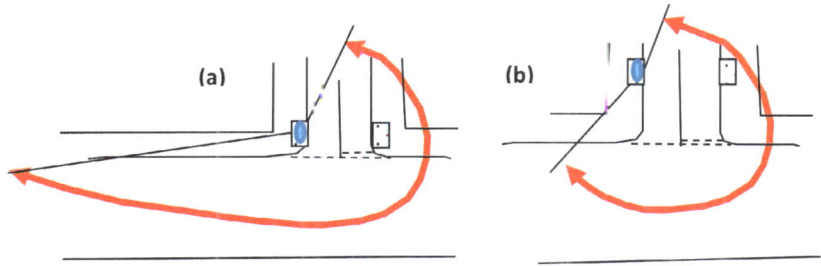

Figure 5.7 Pedestrian's available scanning angle and sight line at junction for crossing at: (a) close to major road, and (b) back from major road.

During this scanning pedestrians must be aware of several key factors which will affect whether to cross or not: first, the Highway Code *specifically* states that if the pedestrian has stepped from the kerb to start crossing, any approaching vehicle turning into the lane into which he or she is moving must give priority. Second, as well as vehicles approaching from behind the pedestrian and turning left into the minor road, this also includes (but is not stated or emphasised in the Highway Code) vehicles approaching from ahead and turning right into the minor road. Third, a vehicle approaching along the minor road toward the junction must give priority to traffic on the major road (Highway Code Rule 172) – presumably, but not stated in the Code, this pedestrian traffic includes people crossing to the left or right of the carriageway.

Thus, pedestrians need to have sufficient time to both turn head and shoulders and see the approaching vehicles. They must then focus and refocus several times in order to judge their speed and evaluate whether the vehicle will obey the Code and accord priority in crossing. The implications of this for the crossing task are that the physical and mental tasks required of pedestrians crossing the minor road are considerable and must be accounted for in the junction's design and layout.

A driver, however, approaching the junction from either direction along the major road, and intending to turn into the minor road, has a much smaller scanning angle, as shown in Figure 5.8, when approaching the junction, requiring minimal head movement and considerably less time before making a decision.

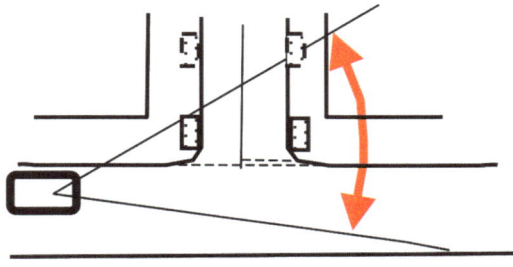

Figure 5.8 Driver scanning angle at a junction

Current Design Guidance: Visibility

Drivers should not be "confused or surprised" when approaching and driving through a junction designed according to the Department for Transport's (DfT's) *Design Manual for Roads and Bridges* (HA/DfT 1992, Part 6; TD 42/95, Chapter 2, Figure 2/1). Consideration is to be made of drivers' need for: horizontal and vertical visibility along the major and minor roads; driveability (i.e. the ease of driving through the junction); smooth vehicular paths; adequate capacity; the ability to see and understand the layout and the path they should follow; and, likely actions of crossing, merging and diverging vehicles.

Pedestrians, however, are not mentioned as needing to avoid "confusion or surprise" when negotiating the junction. Neither is "walkability", similar to the recommended "drivability" for drivers, and neither is "horizontal and vertical visibility along the major and minor roads" nor the "ability to see and understand the path they should follow".

It is recommended, however, to consider the effects on them of different corner radii, guard rails, central refuges and pedestrian crossings, with no suggestions as to specific considerations similar to those for drivers. Guidance states that there should be intervisibility between driver and pedestrian. It appears to be assumed (but is not specifically stated) that intervisibility means that if two moving elements on a potential collision course can see each other, and if either takes action to stop and the other does not, then a collision will be averted. The time or distance of the intervisibility appears to be assumed as the driver's stopping sight distance (SSD), based on the driver's perception-reaction time plus the time for the vehicle to brake to a stop. *Note, however, that the most frequently documented (approximately 70%) causes of vehicle crashes are drivers' inattention (GRCGB 2013), i.e. the vehicle does not slow or stop. This means that for the pedestrian to know that he or she can cross safely, the intervisibility distance should be based on the pedestrian's crossing time,* **not the driver's SSD,** *otherwise the pedestrian cannot be in control of his or her own safety.*

The concepts relating to visibility conditions at a three-way junction are illustrated in Figures 5.9(a), (b) and (c). The car moving at an average speed of 15 mph is about to turn left into the minor arm of the junction where a pedestrian is about to cross. In the 8 sec that the pedestrian needs to walk clear of the car's path the car will have travelled 54 m, which means that the pedestrian must have a sight line towards the car of only 40 m (due to the obstruction of the corner) in order to clear the path of the car if it does not stop.

However, if the pedestrian can only see 15 m beyond the corner, and decides to cross at this designated location, he or she will be crossing without knowing that a potential collision with the approaching car can occur if the driver is distracted or otherwise fails to see him or her. The situation would be particularly severe for a person in a wheelchair or mobility scooter, or a person with a child in a pram, because their line of visibility starts from up to a metre or more from *behind* the kerb, thereby further restricting the distance they can see to approaching vehicles from behind.

PEDESTRIAN TRAFFIC

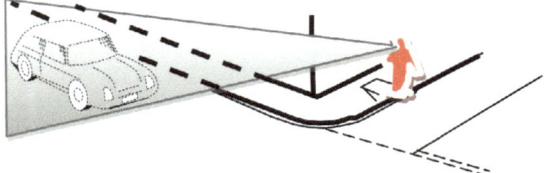

(a) Left-turning car is obscured from pedestrian preparing to cross minor road

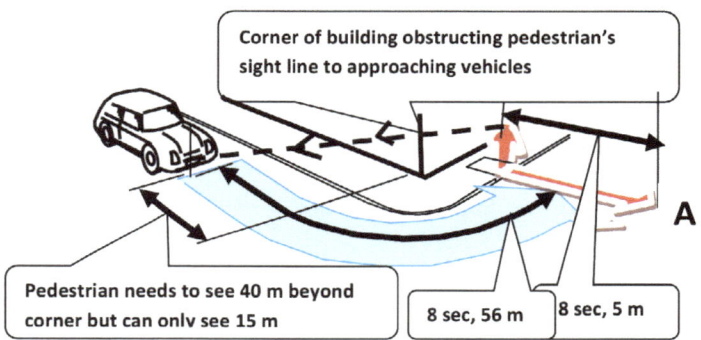

(b) Crossing point defined by ramp several metres from kerbline of major road. In the 8 seconds it takes the pedestrian to walk clear of the car's path (point A, 5 m from the kerb) the car will have travelled 56 m and the pedestrian will have to see 40 m beyond the corner of the building in order to see the car.

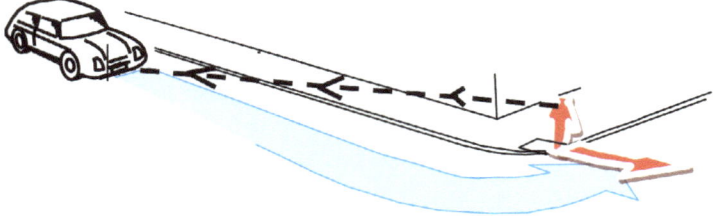

(c) Crossing point defined by ramp close to kerbline of major road. The pedestrian's visibility distance to the approaching car is greater when the crossing point is at the corner. Here, the pedestrian can look back to the approaching car at an adequate distance and can take an informed decision about whether it is safe to cross. Drivers can also better see the pedestrian waiting or starting to cross and can react accordingly in adequate time.

Figure 5.9 Effects of placing pedestrian's crossing point for minor road entrance at corner of footway

Visibility at junctions is recognised from the point of view of drivers, as shown in the sketch of Figure 5.10 (Police Foundation 2013). Here, a driver approaching a junction on the nearside may not be able to see an approaching vehicle on the minor road, or a pedestrian starting to cross when the crossing drop kerb is located back from the main road kerbline. A similar situation can exist when the driver is approaching in the opposite direction and wishes to turn right into the minor road. In both cases, if the driver fails to see the crossing pedestrian a collision is possible.

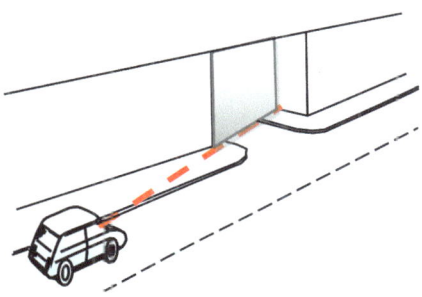

Figure 5.10 Driver's view of minor road junction entrance (Source: Based on Police Foundation 2013)

This emphasises the point illustrated in Figure 5.9, i.e. if the pedestrian's crossing point as designated by the ramp were to be located at the corner, the pedestrian could see a distance that enables an informed decision about whether to start to cross, because his or her sight line distance to the approaching car would be adequate. Alternative solutions could be to lower the speed limit so that approaching vehicles would take longer to reach the crossing point, thereby allowing pedestrians greater time to cross.

An important factor, especially affecting disabled or encumbered pedestrians when crossing, is the ability to take avoiding action if a speeding vehicle suddenly approaches. A disabled person or encumbered pedestrian will be unable to quickly stop and/or reverse direction. Even for a fully aware and able person, however, the need to turn back suddenly when an unexpected vehicle appears in their line of sight can be considered unsafe at best.

Anecdotal evidence indicates that limited sight distances may encourage drivers and pedestrians to be more cautious. Consequently fewer collisions have occurred where sight distances were less than theoretically required. While there is undoubted validity to some aspects of this assertion some considerations include (Schoon 2010):

- Although most drivers may drive more cautiously where there are reduced sight lines, some will drive at a speed which does not enable them to stop in time to avoid a pedestrian who may have looked away from his or her sight line immediately before the approaching vehicle came into view. At the very least the pedestrian will be intimidated and hence reluctant to walk along that route.
- Although greater driver caution due to reduced sight lines may decrease accidents which occur due to the inattention of some pedestrians, this must be weighed against the inconvenience to pedestrians who habitually use caution but are put at risk because of inadequate sight lines.
- For a pedestrian venturing into a situation where reliance must be placed on the driver to avoid a potential collision, a prudent pedestrian cannot allow him- or herself (and accompanying people) to rely on the driver and, for safety's sake, will invariably give priority to the vehicle – a form of intimidation which can lead to a reluctance to walk, especially for disabled or encumbered people. *It should be noted that "Driver/rider failed to look properly" is the most commonly recorded factor in serious and slight accidents (Reported Road Casualties GB 2013).*
- Often, the exercise of caution relies on eye contact between users. This can be unreliable in such cases as poor visibility, tinted windows on vehicles, distracting reflections from the vehicle's windows and, for partially sighted or blind people, the impossibility of making any eye contact.

Layout of Footways Relative to Junction

A further aspect of junction design which may present difficulties for pedestrians is embodied in key elements of *DMRB*. They include the following statement in *DMRB* 5.12:

> Defined at-grade pedestrian crossing points on the minor road should be a minimum of 15 m back from the 'Give Way' line and should be sited so as to reduce to a minimum the width to be crossed by pedestrians provided they are not involved in excessive detours from their desired paths. Central refuges should be used wherever possible, but not in the major road in a rural situation.

In a comment on this guidance Schoon (2015) states:

> However, locating the crossing away from the mouth of the junction (a minimum of 15m back from the 'Give Way' line) conflicts with ways to encourage walking and reduce vehicle speeds. The implied use of large radii kerbs, necessitating the crossing to be back from the Give Way line to reduce the distance to be crossed (and encouraging higher vehicle speeds through the junction), or the use of a central refuge to ease the pedestrian's task of crossing the wider minor road's mouth (but simultaneously increasing the total crossing time and exposure to moving vehicles) are factors which cause further impediments and tasks on pedestrians who wish to cross safely and conveniently.

Consideration could therefore be given to reducing kerb radii and constructing build-outs to reduce pedestrians' crossing distance. This would also necessitate vehicles travelling slower in the major and minor arms of the junction, enable drivers and pedestrians to see each other earlier, give pedestrians shorter time to be exposed to moving vehicles and ensure that pedestrians can maintain their journey along their preferred desire line. The improved visibility of pedestrians would assist approaching drivers in planning speed changes and, therefore, reduce the likelihood of 'shunt'-type collisions between vehicles.

Other aspects of guidance for pedestrians in *DMRB* Volume 6, Section 2 Part 6 TD 42/95 which could benefit from reconsideration with regard to their safety and convenience include:

- Visibility distances should be based on the crossing time and associated distances required by pedestrians and not on the stopping sight distances of approaching vehicles.
- As pedestrians and vehicles are both legally 'traffic' they should be addressed as such in the design remit.
- The width of the typical urban separation island is inadequate (1.5 m).
- The sight lines required by pedestrians are not currently mentioned in the visibility standards.

Regarding provision of guardrails, although it is stated that "the guardrail should not obstruct drivers' visibility requirements" it would also seem prudent for designers to ensure that the guardrail does not impede pedestrians' visibility towards approaching vehicles which, as indicated at the beginning of this chapter, can be a much more complex task, even with a central refuge, than the need for drivers to observe the pedestrians. Of particular importance is the matter of inappropriate positioning or use of a guardrail affecting drivers' visibility of smaller children and people in wheelchairs or on mobility scooters.

Other reasons for providing direct access across a junction in addition to the matter of intervisibility and sight distance addressed earlier include (Schoon 2010):

- In being able to cross directly in line with opposite footways pedestrian traffic, in common with vehicular (including cycle) traffic, the pedestrian can more obviously have priority over

turning vehicles moving along the major road, thereby also assisting compliance with the Highway Code.
- Drivers approaching along the main road from either direction can earlier see pedestrians waiting to cross (or starting to cross) as they approach the junction, than if the pedestrians are obscured by a building corner and/or by vehicles stopped or moving in the junction. This ability of drivers to see pedestrians earlier can therefore enable them to better adjust their actions to permit pedestrians to exercise their priority in crossing.
- In being able to see pedestrians earlier and slowing down in good time, the speed of traffic on the major road is likely to be reduced. This can enhance the effects of speed restrictions and traffic calming, as well as attaining a smoother traffic flow with less likelihood of rear-end collisions.
- Pedestrians are able to see vehicles approaching in the several directions described earlier on the major and minor arms of a junction (up to an angle of 260 degrees) in order for them to evaluate the driver's likely actions and speed before crossing.
- Pedestrians when looking ahead and behind them for approaching vehicles can see a greater distance and therefore are better able to judge if an approaching vehicle is being driven too fast, erratically, or in some other way which appears to pose a threat of collision.
- Pedestrians using mobility scooters equipped with a rear-view mirror are able to see behind them for approaching vehicles on the main road and this may be difficult (and therefore time consuming and uncertain) or impossible if the crossing is not direct.
- Pedestrians are less likely to have to cross between vehicles waiting to exit the minor road. Such a crossing location obscures pedestrians from vehicles turning from the main road, decreases their and drivers' visibility, and can leave the pedestrian in a dangerous position as the vehicular traffic changes. Also, in having to cross at such a location, often defined by the position of dropped kerbs, the pedestrian is forced to

cross between stationary (equivalent to parked) vehicles with engines running, a move specifically warned against in Highway Code Rule 14. For someone either pushing or in a wheelchair, or with a mobility aid, or accompanied by small children, the intimidation, danger and delay in making such a crossing can essentially render their walking journey impossible.
- Pedestrians can cross the carriageway in as short a time as they are able and comfortable.

A more obvious treatment for crossing the minor arm of a priority junction with geometric features which emphasises the pedestrian's priority is that shown in Figure 5.11. This arrangement is also adopted widely in other countries. It has several advantages for pedestrians, including a direct desire line, greater visibility of all vehicle approaches, no obscuration by vehicles during crossing, easier manoeuvrability for wheelchair and scooter users, and less intimidation by turning and stopping vehicles. For drivers it enables the pedestrian to be better seen before and during the pedestrian's crossing, thereby enabling the driver to plan ahead and adjust speed in good time. The carriageway marking also assists pedestrians and drivers in identifying clearly the crossing location.

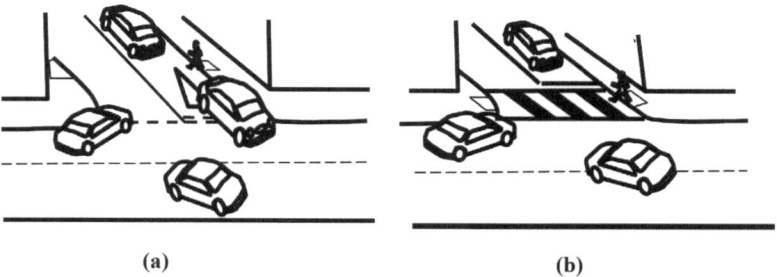

(a) (b)

Figure 5.11 Comparison of current pedestrian crossing arrangements at minor arm of a junction in (a) UK practice and (b) North American practice

A particularly confusing and intimidating situation for pedestrians arises when a traffic island is located on the main arm of a priority junction such that it is unclear whether it should be considered a part of the junction or of the main road. A view of the situation, indicating a vehicle exiting the minor road and turning right into the major road, is shown in the sketches of Figure 5.12. The design options for pedestrians crossing the main road are:

In Figure 5.12(a), one movement straight across in line with the minor arm. Here the pedestrian has priority over the turning vehicle, as indicated in Highway Code Rule 170, "Watch out for pedestrians crossing a road into which you are turning. If they have started to cross they have priority, so give way."

In Figure 5.12(b), one movement several metres from the minor arm. Here it becomes unclear whether the crossing location is a part of the junction and so pedestrians and drivers are unclear about whether the pedestrian has priority in crossing over the vehicle which has turned and is now effectively on a straight segment of carriageway. It should be noted that a pedestrian crossing at any point has priority over vehicles but drivers rarely observe this, and the pedestrian is therefore at risk.

In Figure 5.12(c), potentially two movements across with a central refuge some metres from the minor arm. Accordingly, the driver might assume priority over the pedestrian on the refuge because the turning movement had been completed and the vehicle would now be on a straight segment of carriageway. Therefore, the driver might assume priority over the pedestrian who would be required to wait at the refuge.

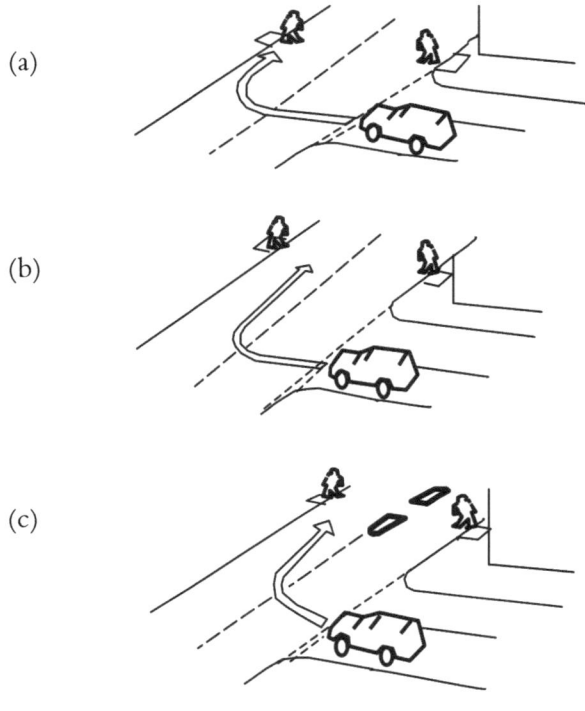

Figure 5.12 Potential confusion of priority movements of vehicles and pedestrians at, and adjacent to, junctions

The above situations would also be repeated substantially in principle for a vehicle turning left from the minor road. It would be preferable if the rules and design guidelines for these crossings at, and adjacent to, junctions were to be clarified. Regardless of the outcome of such investigations a possible arrangement for further exploration could be as shown in the sketch of Figure 5.13. This shows a typical arrangement of a clearly designated pedestrian crossing in which the pedestrians have priority, consistent with Highway Code Rule 170: "Watch out for pedestrians crossing a road into which you are turning. If they have started to cross they have priority, so give way." These are essentially similar to those in many other countries. *Although a criticism of these clear markings is that pedestrians may obtain a 'false sense of security' this would be countered by the clear indications to drivers that pedestrians had priority at these crossings.*

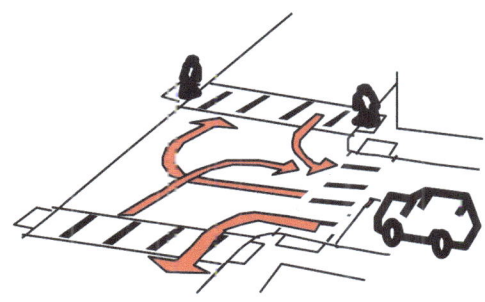

Figure 5.13 Pedestrian crossings typical of many other countries

When a priority junction is configured as a mini roundabout this can pose extremely difficult crossing conditions for pedestrians. The increased speed of vehicles negotiating larger radii corners which sometimes obscure visibility lines, and the lack of any priority for pedestrians at mini roundabouts are major concerns. A potential improvement for pedestrians is shown in Figure 5.14. This shows a marked crossing along a major road with a stop line prior to the actual crossing markings.

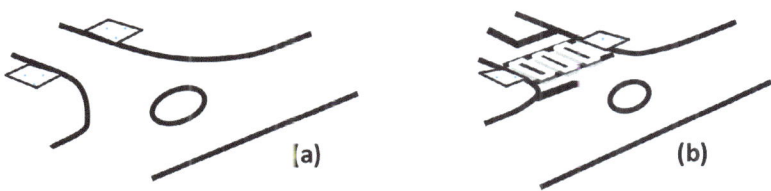

Figures 5.14(a) Current mini roundabout design with no pedestrian priority; (b) potential improved pedestrian crossing showing crossing location and vehicle stop lines

Features of junctions that can improve pedestrians' safety and convenience include:

- reduced corner radii;
- build-outs, the width of which would accommodate the raised table and the length of which, in the direction of crossing, generally would not exceed the typical width of a parallel kerbside parking lane;
- vertical deflections (flat-top humps, speed tables and junction plateaus);
- central refuges (sometimes referred to as islands or separators); and,
- clearly delineated with cross markings.

Potential Modification to Junction Design

To explain the adoption of one or more of these measures consider a priority junction which typically occurs along an urban trunk road with a distributor road. With no central refuge pedestrians have priority over all turning vehicles (left and right turns between the major and minor arms) for the entire width of the minor arm of the carriageway when crossing (Highway Code Rules 170-172). Two factors affect the functioning of the crossing:

- Drivers making turns from the major arms or when approaching the junction along the minor arm often do not observe the pedestrian priority rule and do not stop for pedestrians who have started to cross.
- In UK practice the triangular surface marking superimposed over the pedestrians' route, combined with a stop or yield sign beyond where a pedestrian would cross, would seem to offer a visual deterrent to pedestrians who wish to cross and seems to give drivers no visual clues that pedestrians who have started to cross have priority.

Given the above conditions, one approach to modifying the existing junction or designing a new scheme can be to:

- encourage lower vehicle speeds – by reducing curb radii and installing a raised table at the crossing location, in addition to general lowering of speeds;
- make drivers alert to the need to stop before the crossing location in order to give priority to crossing pedestrians – by installing a raised table, including relevant surface markings and studs if appropriate;
- minimise the crossing distance for pedestrians – by provision of build-outs. This also has the benefit of reducing delay to waiting drivers because pedestrians can clear the crossing faster; and,
- provide an improved sight line to approaching vehicles along the arms of the junction, especially along the minor road, especially where parked vehicles may be present.

Potential changes to the existing layout are shown in Figures 5.15(a) and (b), for example, and contrast considerably with the markings in UK practice which, with the triangular marking superimposed over the pedestrians' route, seem to offer a visual deterrent to crossing.

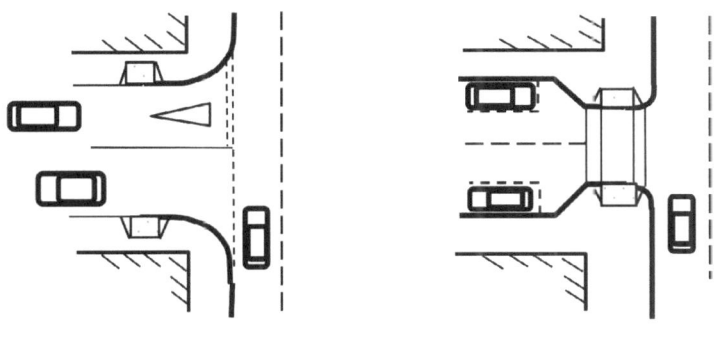

(a) Original priority 3-way junction

(b) Option for maximum narrowing of minor road: build-outs, raised table and reduced radii and parking each side

Figure 5.15 Examples of options in junction design

Regarding a possible solution to pedestrians crossing the entrance to a minor road, the ideal way for both pedestrians and drivers would be to adopt the current convention that a turning vehicle gives priority to traffic approaching in the opposite direction. Since pedestrians are traffic, *this rule should apply to pedestrians seen approaching the crossing location of a junction as well as when they have actually started crossing when there is a risk of collision with the turning vehicle – as is the case with approaching vehicles.*

Particular difficulties may be experienced by mobility scooter users at junctions, as shown in Figure 5.16, and advantages of locating the crossing 'in line' are that the scooter and other users have improved sight lines to oncoming vehicles. Ease of looking behind may be improved (but not necessarily fully relied upon) by the use of handlebar mirrors on the scooter (Schoon 2010).

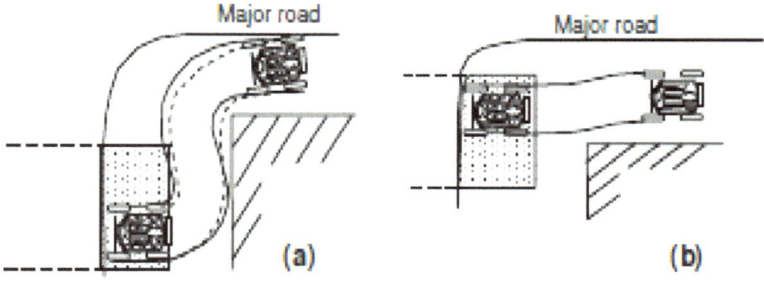

Figure 5.16 Illustrative comparison of four-wheeled mobility scooter trajectory for a minor road junction crossing located (a) some distance from the major road and (b) in line with opposite footway

A particular form of raised table is the side raised entry treatment (SRET). Side entry treatments are road sections at junctions of side roads with major roads. They are placed either at the entrance to the junction or within a short distance of it. Based on a study by Buchanan and Associates (ca 1995) and a more detailed investigation by Wood et al. (2006), TfL (2007) posed the following research questions:

1. Are SRETs beneficial to pedestrians' safety on the feature itself?
2. Are SRETs beneficial to road safety at the junction and on the side road?

SRETs have been installed to achieve a combination of objectives (e.g. TfL streetscape guidance) including:

- creating a strong visual threshold for traffic leaving or entering a minor road;
- providing easier pedestrian movement by raising treatment;
- assisting pedestrian priority;
- deterring parking close to junctions;
- slowing vehicle speeds; and,
- reducing collisions involving vulnerable road users.

The findings suggest that SRETs do provide easier pedestrian movement and assist pedestrians in asserting priority. The findings further indicate that SRETs reduce collisions involving pedal cycles.

In terms of general layout, crossroads are convenient for pedestrians, as they minimise diversion from desire lines when crossing the street (*MfS 2007*). Although staggered junctions can reduce vehicle conflict compared with crossroads, they reduce directness for pedestrians. If potential user conflict exists, consideration may be given to replacing the junction on a speed table, or closing one of the arms to motor traffic.

Signalised and Other Crossing Locations

So far, the discussion has focused on junctions and primarily on the location of crossing points related to the pedestrian's sight lines to approaching vehicles. The necessity for pedestrians to see approaching vehicles at a sufficient distance to cross safely has been stressed, together with physical features of the junction which facilitate this.

Recognition of the need for a review of pedestrians walking speeds (and, hence crossing times) is addressed by Crabtree, et al (2014) in which it is concluded that: more research is needed to determine the economic benefits of greater clearance times which enable people to cross; the assumed 1.2 m/s walking speed cannot be achieved by many people; the cost of walking is less than that of driving and pedestrians should be included in all cost appraisals; more Puffin crossings, which can extend maximum periods if necessary, should be installed; greater use of 'countdown' signalised crossings should be made, to assist pedestrians in deciding whether to start to cross; and, clearance times should be increased to assist pedestrians who walk slower than the assumed 1.2 m/s. Further, use of technological improvements to vary the available crossing times and investigations on the effects on safety are also recommended.

Similar principles and concepts related to junctions also apply to crossings in general. In such cases a pedestrian's sight distance may be restricted because of a bend or bends in the road, and driveways or side roads from which an emerging vehicle is obscured near a pedestrian's convenient or essential crossing point. Other obstructions such as parked vehicles or street furniture may present similar problems.

Example of a Crossing Problem and Potential Solutions

A practical case may illustrate a sight distance problem for pedestrians. This involves a situation in Heswall, Wirral (Wirral Pedestrian Association website 2014), where a convenient and essential crossing point is located on a road with nearby bends. In this case, the pedestrian's time to cross was measured and recorded as 11 sec. For a vehicle travelling at 30 mph (12 m/sec) and not slowing or stopping, the pedestrian would need a sight distance to just cross safely of:

> 11 sec x 12 m/sec = 121 m in order to cross just as a vehicle reached the crossing point.

If, however, a 2-sec safety margin were allowed, the required distance would be:
(11 + 2) sec x 12 m/sec = 156 m.

However, the pedestrian's actual sight distance at this point is only 80 m – dangerously less than the 156 m calculated above. Clearly, some review of the traffic regulations and facilities would appear to be advisable and /or a reduced speed limit would appear to be appropriate.

★

Numerous junctions, crossing layouts and speed/sight line locations, visibility and detail dimensions are dangerous for pedestrians and force motorists to risk collisions with them. Regarding design analysis, it must be recognised that for safety: pedestrian capabilities must reflect those described in Chapter 2; pedestrians' sight distances must be greater than a driver's stopping sight distance (SSD); a major reason for collisions is drivers not seeing pedestrians, therefore reliance on drivers stopping for pedestrians who are crossing cannot be the criteria for safe design as at present; and the matter of 'intervisibility' between drivers and pedestrians needs greater examination and clearer definition of the relative approach times and distances between drivers and pedestrians. In the physical layout of junctions and bends: improvements to the definition of crossing locations; reduction of crossing widths by build-outs and often assisted by reduced corner radii; positioning of drop kerbs to reflect desire lines; and installation of raised surfaces can all assist in easing pedestrians' movement and safety. Coordination in the design process between the requirements of the Green Cross Code of the Highway Code regarding users' priorities, and dynamic movement characteristics of pedestrians as well as vehicles also needs to be undertaken. Design procedures sensitive to pedestrians and other users must be established.

References

Berrymans Lace Mawer (2008) *Pedestrian Claims*. Motor Claims Update_MGB, PNG, PEN_(RAW, ACH) 11/08. London.

Colin Buchanan and Associates (ca 1995). *Justification and Design of Entry Treatments*. Assessment Study for the London Transport Director. London.

Crabtree, M., Lodge, C., Emmerson, P. (2014) *A Review of Pedestrian Walking Speeds and Time Needed to Cross the Road*. Transport Research Laboratory, prepared for Living Streets, London.

Department for Transport (Latest Date) *Design Manual for Roads and Bridges* (HA/DfT 1992, Part 6; TD 42/95, Chapter 2, Figure 2/1).

Department for Transport/Driver and Vehicle Licensing Agency (2015) *The Highway Code*. London.

Legislation UK gov.com (2004) *Traffic Management Act Part 2, Section 31*. London.

Police Foundation/Stationery Office (2013) *Roadcraft. The Police Driver's Handbook*. London.

Schoon, John G. (2010) *Mobility Scooters and User Characteristics at Crossings and Intersections*. TRANSED conference proceedings, Montreal 2010.

Schoon, John G. (2010) *Pedestrian Facilities: Engineering and Geometric Design*. Thomas Telford, London.

Transport for London (2007) *Effect of Side Road Entry Treatment on Road Safety in London. London Road Safety Unit Research Summary No. 9*. London.

Wirral Pedestrian Association (2014) *Street Audit – Dawstone Road, Gayton, Wirral – 22 September 2014.* Website accessed December 2015.

Wood, K., Crinson, L.F. and Castle, J.A. (2006) *Effect of Side Raised Entry Treatments for Road Safety in London.* Published project report. TRL, Crowthorne.

CHAPTER 6

THE HIGHWAY CODE

Advice, ambiguity and omissions

The purpose of the Highway Code is to interpret and communicate highway laws for road users. Such interpretation and communication often in practice make it difficult for pedestrians to walk conveniently and safely. Particularly when the Code affects priority of movement of different users, its rules should be comprehensive, clear and unambiguous, but often they are none of these. In reality, neither the rules nor their interpretation by road users result in a fail-safe operating system. Many of the Code's illustrations are aimed primarily at drivers and often do not also show pedestrian crossings, drop-kerbs and marking, and so de-emphasise many features important to all traffic modes operating in unison. Here we look at some of the key features where the Code may be questioned and improvements considered, particularly from the perspective of pedestrians' safety and convenience.

★

The importance of the Highway Code is well recognised in helping compliance with the rules and regulations designed to ensure road safety. The Code (Driving Standards Agency (DSA) 2015) also provides a list of Acts and Regulations which form a legal basis for the Code itself.

As stated in the introduction to the Highway Code:

> Knowing and applying the rules contained in the Highway Code could significantly reduce road casualties. Cutting the

number of deaths and injuries that occur on our roads every year is a responsibility we all share.

But despite this 'code of conduct' road users do not always follow the instructions – either knowingly, through error, or through confusion about its meaning.

Design of pedestrian features of highways as given by governmental advice and guidance, should, of course, show awareness of the movements of road users and vehicles in accordance with the Code's instructions. However, the Code is not mentioned in official design guidelines such as the *Manual for Streets (MfS 2007)* or the *Design Manual for Roads and Bridges (DMRB)* – the major sources of guidance on road and street design. Neither is there mention in the design manuals, for example, of the time and movements needed by pedestrians when they start and cross a road in accordance with the Code's instructions.

Establishing rules and channelling pedestrians' movements in order for them to be 'safe', and which may minimise legal liability in case of accidents, appears to have been the predominant aim of the Highway Code. As quoted by the Commission for Architecture and the Built Environment (CABE) (2002): "The deficiencies in the Code, the lack of compliance by some road users, and the response of official agencies and institutions in establishing guidance complicate the task of designing for pedestrians." CABE's response:

> Recommendation 12: the Highway Code should be rewritten to place greater emphasis on the multiple use of streets, rather than mainly vehicle movement.
>
> Also, the Highway Code is "… addressed mainly at drivers and says little about what are the rights and duties of pedestrians. Pedestrians are confused about what they can and cannot do, which only increases their sense of vulnerability on the street".

Some specific areas where the Code may need re-examination regarding crossing generally are as follows (Schoon 2010):

> Instructions to pedestrians related to central islands (refuges), which are often important for pedestrians when crossing, seem in some respects illogical. Several areas where greater clarity could be beneficial include:
>
> - The rationale for why a pedestrian who has started to cross at a zebra crossing or uncontrolled crossing with a central island must treat the second half of their crossing as a separate crossing is not apparent. This would seem to be a case where time delays for motorists are considered more valuable than for pedestrians, who often have to wait on the island due to vehicles approaching on the second half of the crossing.
> - It is not stated in the Code that if a central refuge is provided at the crossing of the minor arm of a junction this means that the pedestrian must treat the crossing as a single movement or as two separate movements. The latter case would negate a pedestrian's priority (if indeed this is the case) over the entire length of the crossing if a central island is not present, and is a matter for confusion.

In view of the above points several areas of further investigation appear warranted to assist in designing pedestrian facilities which can, by their configuration and dimensions, improve the safety and convenience of all road users. They include:

- the nature of change in pedestrians' crossing priorities brought about by use of central islands (refuges); and,
- clarification of rules about priorities at central islands resulting from their location and function, including free-standing, uncontrolled, zebra, signalled, mid-block and junction.

Pedestrians are covered in the Code's section on "vulnerable road users" but the location and nature of the care is far less detailed or specific as when, for example, the driver is turning across a traffic stream and is instructed to avoid other vehicles. This may account for the confusion and danger where drivers appear not to be aware that they must accord priority to pedestrians. The general statement for drivers to "look out for pedestrians and cyclists" is insufficiently specific in this respect. The expression 'look out for' is not the same as 'give priority to'.

In some specific cases where drivers' actions are addressed, pedestrians are ignored as part of the total driving situation and addressed separately in different, less definitive rules. This fragments the advice and so, in the portions addressed to drivers, pedestrians could be construed as incidental to the total driving task instead of being an essential part of all traffic.

Furthermore, it is often not stated how the extra care is to be given, rather than the more definitive advice to drive or to "give priority to". In addition to the rules about crossing at designated places mentioned above, much attention is devoted to the movement of traffic, including pedestrian traffic, at junctions, including roundabouts. Rules where information for road users could be more informative and assist the safety and convenience of pedestrians are examined on a rule-by-rule basis below. The initial comments made by the author and have been reviewed by the Department for Transport (DfT 2015). These responses are reflected in the author's comments to each rule.

The various aspects of the Code which appear to need immediate attention are addressed by:

- A **description** of the Code's rule.
- An **observation** by the author on the deficiency related to pedestrians' interests.
- **Comments** by the author on possible considerations in which

the Code could be improved. These reflect a review by DfT (Doyle/DfT 2015) on the author's initial observations.

Rule 7: The Green Cross Code. "The advice given below on crossing the road is for all pedestrians. Children should be taught the Code and should not be allowed out alone until they can understand and use it properly. The age when they can do this is different for each child. Many children cannot judge how fast vehicles are going or how far away they are. Children learn by example, so parents and carers should always use the Code in full when out with their children. They are responsible for deciding at what age children can use it safely by themselves.

"A. First find a safe place to cross and where there is space to reach the pavement on the other side. Where there is a crossing nearby, use it. It is safer to cross using a subway, a footbridge, an island, a Zebra, Pelican, Toucan or Puffin crossing, or where there is a crossing point controlled by a police officer, a school crossing patrol or a traffic warden. Otherwise choose a place where you can see clearly in all directions. Try to avoid crossing between parked cars (see Rule 14), on a blind bend, or close to the brow of a hill. Move to a space where drivers and riders can see you clearly. Do not cross the road diagonally."

Observation and Comment*: A safe and convenient place to cross cannot always be found (often at provided drop kerbs) where he or she has an adequate sight line to approaching vehicles. Pedestrian sight lines are not considered adequately in design of junctions and other places where obstructions exist. 'Intervisibility' in the design of junctions does not adequately address pedestrians' capabilities.*

Rule 8: At a junction. "When crossing the road, look out for traffic turning into the road, especially from behind you. If you have started crossing and traffic wants to turn into the road, you have priority and they should give way." (See also comments for Rule 170).

Observation and Comment:
- *The comment for Rule 7A, above, also applies here.*
- *Pedestrians also have priority over vehicles:*
  - *approaching in front of them and turning right across their path;*
  - *along the road on which they are crossing (the minor road on a T junction).*

… and it would seem appropriate to inform pedestrians of this and also to so inform drivers in Rule 170 and rules affecting places where pedestrians cross.

Rule 19: Zebra crossings. "Give traffic plenty of time to see you and to stop before you start to cross. Vehicles will need more time when the road is slippery. Wait until traffic has stopped from both directions or the road is clear before crossing. Remember that traffic does not have to stop until someone has moved onto the crossing. Keep looking both ways, and listening, in case a driver or rider has not seen you and attempts to overtake a vehicle that has stopped."

Observation: *This rule as stated is contradictory. The pedestrian cannot wait for traffic to stop at the same time as stepping into the carriageway to make it stop.*

Comment: *Consider modifying the Code to state that vehicles should stop when a pedestrian is waiting on the footway to cross.*

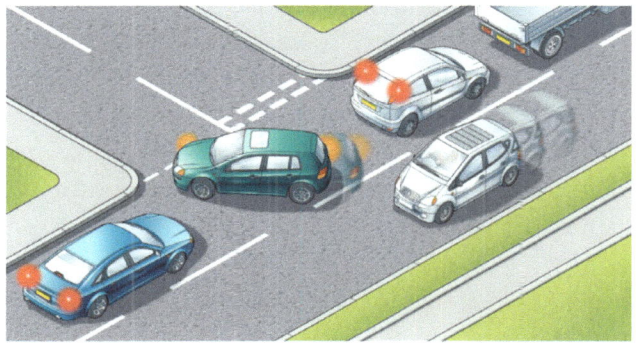

Rule 151: Do not block access to a side road

Rule 151: In slow-moving traffic. You should: "… be aware of cyclists and motorcyclists who may be passing on either side".

Observation: Should drivers be aware also of crossing pedestrians who may not have safe places to cross? Also, the diagram titled "Do not block access to a side road" in this section does not show pedestrian facilities or pedestrians who may also be crossing the minor road entrance.

Comment: The location clearly shows a major road along which pedestrians are likely to walk, with a requirement to cross the mouth of the minor road in both directions. Many junctions of this type exist and need to be crossed safely. Illustrating the appropriated drop kerbs and a pedestrian crossing the intersecting road would help drivers to be aware of this possibility.

Rule 163: Overtake only when it is safe and legal to do so. You should: "… not get too close to the vehicle you intend to overtake. Give motorcyclists, cyclists and horse riders at least as much room as you would when overtaking a car".

Observation: Pedestrians are just as likely to be crash victims as motorcyclists, horse riders or cyclists.

Comment: Why not give pedestrians the extra care by mentioning them in the rule in whatever situation they are likely to be injured? This rule should also include overtaking of pedestrians when there is no footway, such as along a rural road and along segments of roads where the footway is too rough or inadequate and pedestrians are forced to walk along the carriageway.

Rule 170: Take extra care at junctions. You should: "… watch out for pedestrians crossing a road into which you are turning. If they have started to cross they have priority, so give way".

Observation: There are eight different combinations of vehicle and pedestrian movements for a simple T junction (see Figures 6.1 and 6.2) where only one is shown diagrammatically in the Code.

Comment: *This rule needs much more emphasis for drivers on each of the possible turning movements, including diagrams of each of the circumstances.*

It should also take note of the comments below for Rules 171, 172 and 206.

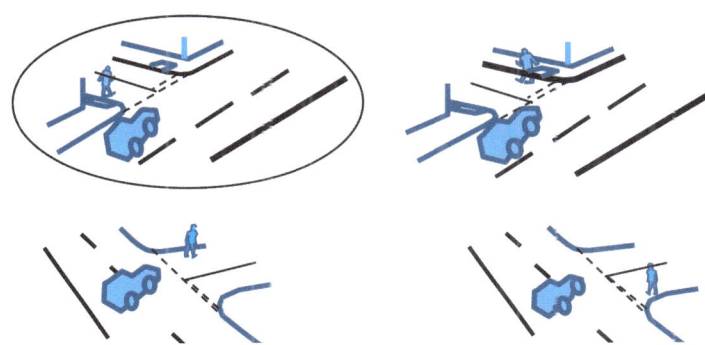

Figure 6.1 Pedestrian priority over turning vehicles at three-way priority junctions – pedestrian crossing minor arm of junction. Only the situation circled is shown in the Highway Code.

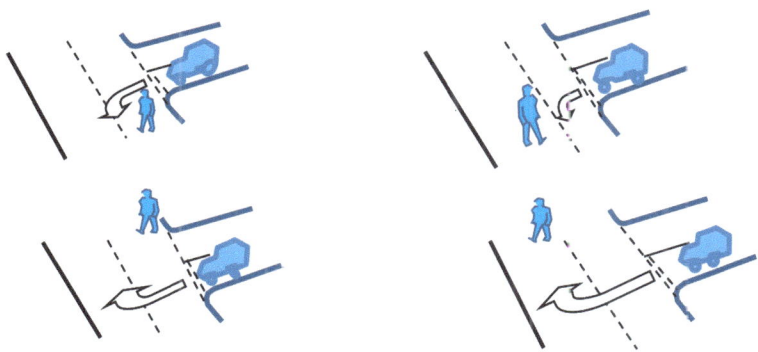

Figure 6.2 Pedestrian priority over turning vehicles at three-way priority junctions – pedestrian crossing major arms of the junction. None of these situations is illustrated in the Highway Code.

PEDESTRIAN TRAFFIC

Rule 171. "You **MUST** stop behind the line at a junction with a 'Stop' sign and a solid white line across the road. Wait for a safe gap in the traffic before you move off." (Laws RTA 1988 sect 36 & TSRGD regs 10 & 16).

Rule 172. "The approach to a junction may have a 'Give Way' sign or a triangle marked on the road. You **MUST** give way to traffic on the main road when emerging from a junction with broken white lines across the road." (Laws RTA 1988 sect 36 & TSRGD regs 10(1), 16(1) & 25).

Observation: *In Rules 171 and 172 it is not clear that a pedestrian crossing the minor road parallel to the major road must be accorded priority over vehicles approaching the junction along the minor road, as shown in Figure 6.3. Rule 171 states to drivers: "Wait for a safe gap in the traffic before you move off." Therefore, because pedestrians are defined as 'traffic' (Traffic Management Act 2004, Section 31) it would seem to be logical and appropriate that priority of pedestrians over vehicles approaching on the minor road should be clearly stated.*

Comment: *Again, it is not stated **how** pedestrians are to be given extra care. Preferably this rule should state that the vehicles stop before the stop line and also clear of pedestrians crossing because the objective of this is to assist users in using the roads safely.*

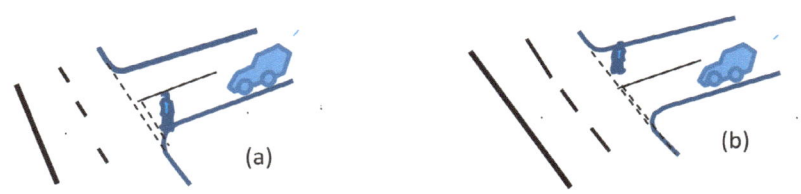

Figure 6.3 Priority of a pedestrian crossing the mouth of a minor road (a) left of vehicle to right, (b) right of vehicle to left. Neither is mentioned or shown in the Highway Code.

Rule 206. Drive carefully and slowly when: "… turning at road junctions; give way to pedestrians who are already crossing the road into which you are turning".

Observation: *When it is stated that pedestrians have priority in these cases several other situations arise which are not illustrated in the Code and which would better inform drivers about what is required.*

Comment: *Such illustrations would indicate that pedestrians have priority also crossing the arms being turned into on the major road at a junction as well as at the minor arm. The diagrams shown earlier in Figures 6.1, 6.2 and 6.3 illustrate this point.*

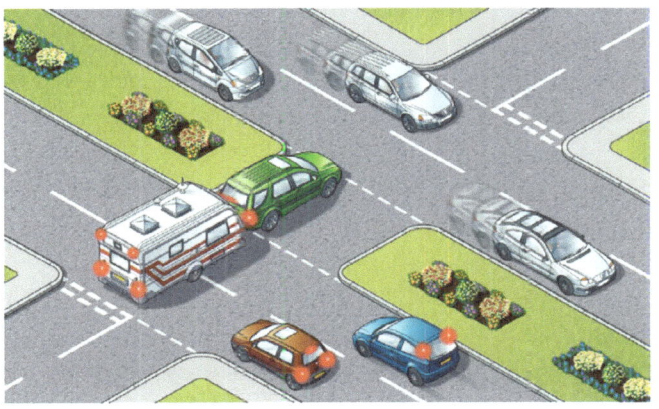

Rule 173: Assess your vehicle's length and do not obstruct traffic

Rule 173: Dual carriageways

Observation: *The illustration titled "Assess your vehicle's length and do not obstruct traffic" shows no pedestrian facilities. Although these are not the focus of the illustration, their omission diminishes the importance of pedestrian facilities throughout the road network.*

Comment: *Rules for pedestrians also directly affect drivers. Awareness and coordination of drivers' actions could be improved by including pedestrian facilities on the illustration.*

PEDESTRIAN TRAFFIC

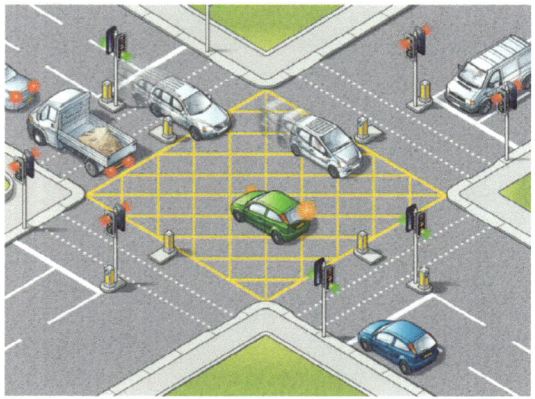

Rule 174: Enter a box junction only if your exit road is clear

Rule 174: Box Junctions. "These have criss-cross yellow lines painted on the road. You **MUST NOT** enter the box…"

Observation: It should also be stated that drivers should be stopped by pedestrians crossing the road into which the vehicle is turning – pedestrians crossing should be shown on the illustration.

Comment: Despite the advice in Rule 170, and its accompanying photo, the advice to drivers is incomplete and therefore dangerous from a pedestrian collision point of view.

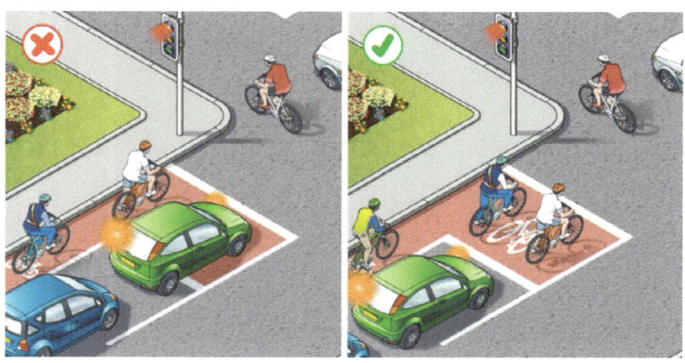

Rule 178: Do not unnecessarily encroach on the cyclists' waiting area

Rule 178: Advanced stop lines (Laws RTA 188 sect 36 & TSRG regs. 10,36(1) & 43(2)).

Observation: *The illustrations titled "Do not unnecessarily encroach on the cyclists' waiting area" shows no pedestrian facilities. Although these are not the focus of the illustrations, their omission diminishes the importance of pedestrian facilities throughout the road network.*

Comment: *Rules for pedestrians also directly affect drivers. Awareness and coordination of drivers' actions could be improved by including pedestrian facilities on the illustration.*

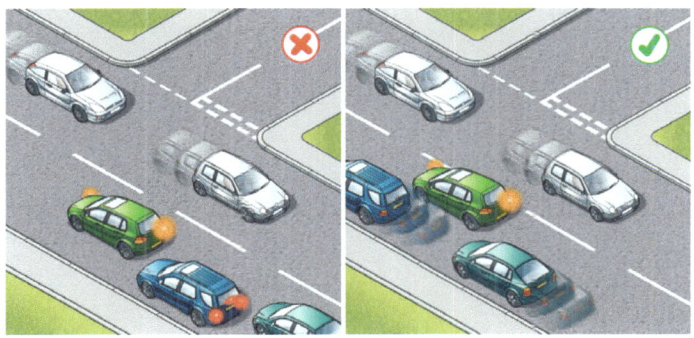

Rule 180: Position your vehicle correctly to avoid obstructing traffic

Rule 180: Turning right. "Wait until there is a safe gap between you and any oncoming vehicle. Watch out for cyclists, motorcyclists, pedestrians and other road users".

Observation: *No pedestrians or pedestrian facilities are mentioned or shown in the illustration for this rule.*

Comment: *"Watch out for" is not sufficient. Although pedestrian crossing facilities are shown in Rules for Pedestrians, this is a critical location where the rule applies to drivers also and is essential for safe crossing of pedestrians. Pedestrian crossing facilities, pedestrians and other road users should be shown in the critical locations of the illustration.*

PEDESTRIAN TRAFFIC

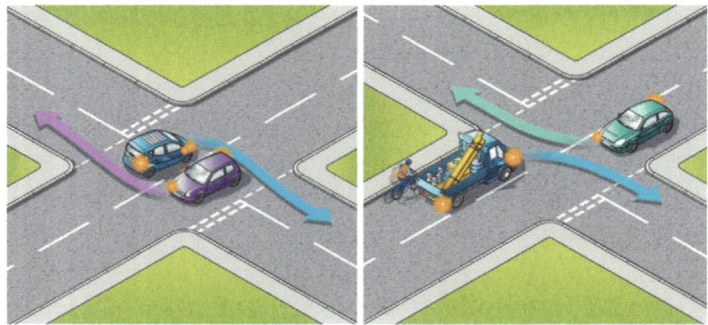

Rule 181: Left – Turning right side to right side. Right – Turning left side to left side

Rule 181: "When turning right at crossroads where an oncoming vehicle is also turning right, there is a choice of two methods:

- Turn right side to right side; keep the other vehicle on your right and turn behind it. This is generally the safer method as you have a clear view of any approaching traffic when completing your turn.
- Left side to left side, turning in front of each other. This can block your view of oncoming vehicles, so take extra care. Cyclists and motorcyclists in particular may be hidden from your view…"

Observation: No pedestrians, who may also be blocked from view, or pedestrian facilities, are shown in the illustration for this rule.

Comment: More than requiring extra care, they need to be accorded priority and it would be desirable to state that pedestrians may also be blocked from view. This should be clearly stated, especially where turning vehicles cross the parts of the junction where they have priority. Also, no pedestrian crossing facilities are indicated in the illustrations for this rule and it would be advisable to show them.

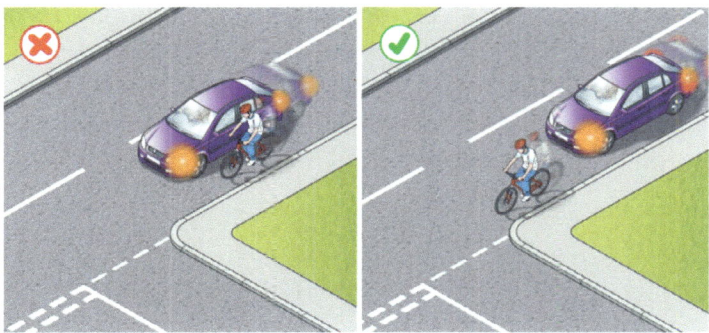

Rule 182: Do not cut in on cyclists

Rule 182: Turning left. "Cyclists, motorcyclists and other road users in particular may be hidden from your view".

Observation*: So will pedestrians and this should be specifically stated. In the illustration for this rule no pedestrian facilities are shown although the left-turning vehicle must give way to pedestrians crossing the minor arm of the junction illustrated. This case is so obvious that pedestrian facilities should be described and shown.*

DfT response to author: *This point is covered in Rule 170 but we can consider specifically adding pedestrians here when the Code is next revised.*

Rule 183 (no picture): "When turning:

- keep as close to the left as is safe and practicable;
- give way to any vehicles using a bus lane, cycle lane or tramway from either direction".

Observation*: Also, the pedestrian crossing should be shown and 'give way to crossing pedestrians' should be noted.*

Comment*: This rule is incomplete. Drivers must make decisions based on multiple simultaneous traffic movement conditions of which pedestrians are* *an essential part and as important as 'any vehicle'. The fact that Rule 170 also applies does not lessen the importance of this multiple, simultaneous traffic movement. Note that rules should complement and reinforce each other not replace them. Preferably, add to this rule in the second item, "cyclists, motorcyclists and other road users".*

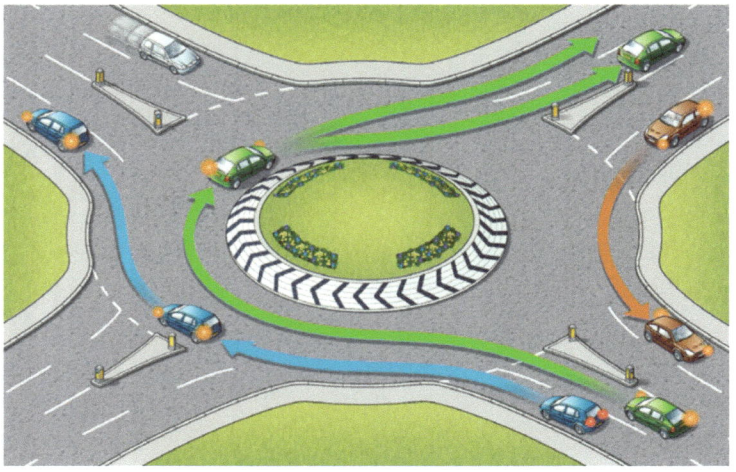

Rule 185: Follow the correct procedure at roundabouts

Rule 185: "When reaching the roundabout you should:

- give priority to traffic approaching from your right, unless directed otherwise by signs, road markings or traffic lights
- check whether road markings allow you to enter the roundabout without giving way. If so, proceed, but still look to the right before joining
- watch out for all other road users already on the roundabout; be aware they may not be signalling correctly or at all
- look forward before moving off to make sure traffic in front has moved off."

Observation*: All of these instructions emphasise looking to the right and ignore the fact that a pedestrian may have started to cross from the left before* the vehicle reaches the 'Give Way' line. This is one of the serious deficiencies of roundabouts and it would seem advisable to inform drivers to also look to the left for pedestrians.

Comment: *The illustration for this rule titled "Follow the correct procedure at roundabouts" gives no indication that pedestrians or their crossing needs exist, and it would be desirable to advise drivers to look for pedestrians from the left as well as looking to the right for vehicles. The illustration should show marked pedestrian crossings and pedestrians since they are part of "all other road users".*

Rule 187 (no picture): Roundabout. "In all cases watch out for and give plenty of room to pedestrians who may be crossing the approach and exit roads…"

Observation: *Similar to that for Rule 185, above.*

Comment: *More than "watch out for", it would be advisable to specifically state that pedestrians have priority if already crossing the carriageway on a potential collision course.*

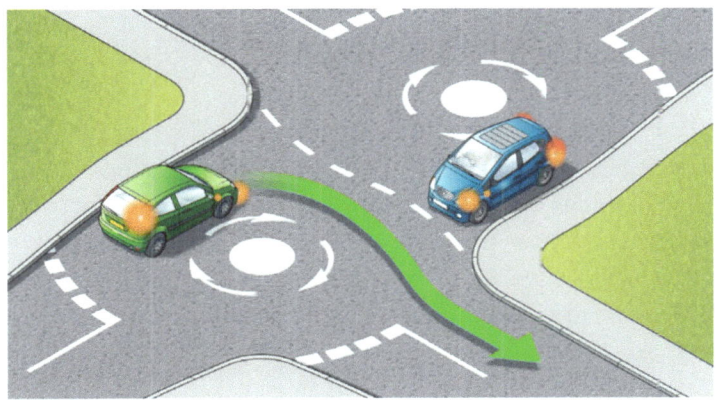

Rule 190: Treat each roundabout separately

Rule 188: Mini roundabouts (Laws RTA 1988 sect 36 & TSRGD regs 10(1) & 16(1)). "Approach these in the same way as normal roundabouts".

Observation*: The same deficiencies exist in the Highway Code with respect to pedestrians as for Rule 186. There is again no indication in the illustration for this section on mini roundabouts showing pedestrian facilities and how drivers should behave in terms of right of way.*

Comment*: Because mini roundabouts are common features of urban road networks, this is a serious omission and it would be advisable to address pedestrians' needs both in the text and by illustration.*

Concluding Remarks

Many areas of ambiguity, apparent inconsistency, partial information and selective provision of information exist in what otherwise is an essential and in many cases informative document.

Much of the lack of clarity in the Code reportedly may encourage road users to be more cautious. This caution is particularly relevant in the case of priority. Here, a vulnerable road user's insistence of right of way or lack of observation, combined with a driver's lack of attention or error, could result in a collision.

Lack of clarity, however, can cause confusion. This, in the event of driver/pedestrian interaction, can be equally dangerous. Also, the degree of additional caution which pedestrians must exercise can significantly detract from the utility, convenience and, therefore, attractiveness of walking. To improve the Code and assure that its provisions lead to greater safety and convenience for all road users, it will be essential that policies and practices in users' education, enforcement and conduct also be addressed.

★

> The Code is based upon Acts and Regulations which have evolved over the years. It was initially devised to respond to the increased popularity of motor vehicles. This may partially explain that whereas the Code is quite complete in illustrating all of the situations where vehicle-to-vehicle interaction can occur, it is deficient in illustrating the many situations involving vehicles and pedestrians. Consequently, matters of pedestrian movement and priority locations, many of them illustrated in this chapter, have been examined. It will be essential to closely co-ordinate the instructions, priorities and movement of vehicles and pedestrians as described in the Code with the design of junctions and other crossings if the full benefits of the Code are to be obtained.

References

CABE (2002) *Paving the Way*. London.

Department for Transport/Driving Standards Agency (2015) *The Highway Code*. London.

Department for Transport (2004) Traffic Management Act 2004, Section 31, *Network Management Duty Guidance*. London.

Department for Transport (2015) Response dated 5 May 2015 to queries by J.G. Schoon.

Schoon J.G. (2010) *Pedestrian Facilities: Geometric Design and Engineering*. Thomas Telford, London.

CHAPTER 7

SPEED, ALCOHOL and INEXPERIENCE

Carnage and opportunity

High speed, too much alcohol and inexperience of young drivers feature in about 30% of all road casualties – killing and maiming not only the people responsible but others, including pedestrians of all ages and abilities. Also, drunk pedestrians contribute to their own deaths and injuries. Yet we haven't made much improvement despite the now ample evidence of why and how drivers speed and drink to excess, and how their inexperience contributes to collisions. Recognising the difficulties and possibilities for change is a first and essential step; the Royal Society for the Prevention of Accidents (RoSPA) and others such as the Institute for Advanced Motorists (IAM) have long investigated these concerns. Speeding issues focus on the effectiveness of cameras, enforcement, education, vehicle adaptation and road engineering. Alcohol abuse is addressed in terms of its availability, limits, penalties, remedial action and vehicle modifications. Numerous organisations are concerned with reducing the casualties caused by inexperience, mainly by introduction of the Graduated Licensing Scheme (GLS). Key features of RoSPA's findings and recommendations, as well as from other concerned authors, focusing on involvement of pedestrians, are outlined here.

★

SPEEDING

Inappropriate Speed

Inappropriate speed includes both exceeding the speed limit and driving or riding within the speed limit when this is too fast for the conditions, such as poor weather or high pedestrian activity (RoSPA 2011). Inappropriate speed contributes to around 14% of all injury collisions, 15% of crashes resulting in a serious injury and 24% of collisions which result in a death and are recorded by the police (Department for Transport (DfT) 2011).

Higher speeds are more likely to result in crashes and more severe injuries to drivers and other road users. These speeds also magnify other driver errors, such as driving when tired or distracted, so increasing the chances of causing a collision. Some important aspects of speeding include (RoSPA 2011):

- Drivers' recognition of, and reaction to, danger requires a greater distance travelled before action is taken, and the vehicle takes longer to stop.
- Around two-thirds of crashes in which people are killed or injured occur on roads with a speed limit of 30 mph or less.
- At 30 mph vehicles are travelling at 44 ft (about three car lengths) each second. One blink and the driver may fail to see a child emerge from behind a parked car.
- Even in good conditions, the difference in stopping distance between 30 mph and 35 mph is an extra 21 ft, more than two car lengths.
- A 1 mph reduction in average speed would reduce accident frequency by about 6% on urban main roads and 4% on residential roads with low average speeds.
- Drivers who speed are more likely to be involved in collisions. They are also more likely to commit other driving violations, such as red-light running and driving too close.

Speed and Safety

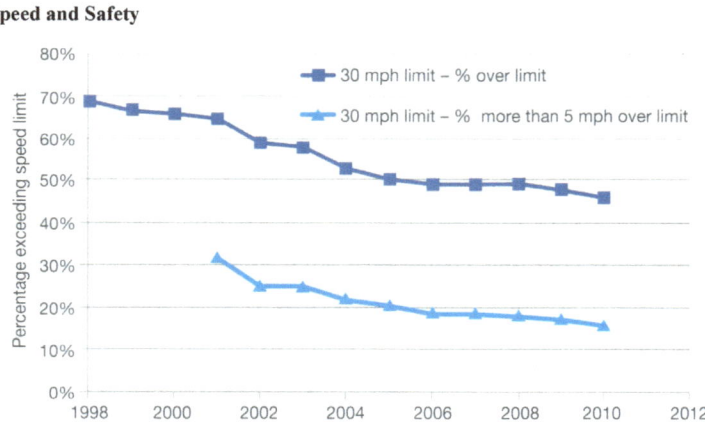

Figure 7.1 Percentage of cars exceeding the 30 mph speed limit and the limit plus 5 mph on built-up roads (Source: Mitchell 2012, Fig. 2)

In recent years, speeds have come down. These and associated trends and correlations described below were analysed and reported by Mitchell (2012). Figure 7.1 shows the percentage of cars on built-up roads that exceed the speed limit and, since 2001, the limit plus 5 mph on 30 mph roads in free-flow conditions. The reduction in cars exceeding the limit on 30 mph roads fell from 69% in 1998 to 46% in 2010. The percentage exceeding the limit by more than 5 mph is much lower, and has proportionally declined from 32% in 2001 to 16% in 2010. The average speed reduced from 32 mph in 2001 to 29.8 mph in 2010 (about 7%). These trends have continued at approximately the same rate since 2010.

Pedestrians are about 40% of all fatalities on built-up roads, and the severity of injury is known to be particularly affected by the speed of vehicles. In 2010, 81% of pedestrians injured in urban areas were hit by cars, as were 68% of pedestrian fatalities (DfT, 2011).

The reduction in speeding offences and the reduction in speeds that would normally trigger offences could be due to an increasing number of drivers taking speed awareness courses instead of having points added to their licence.

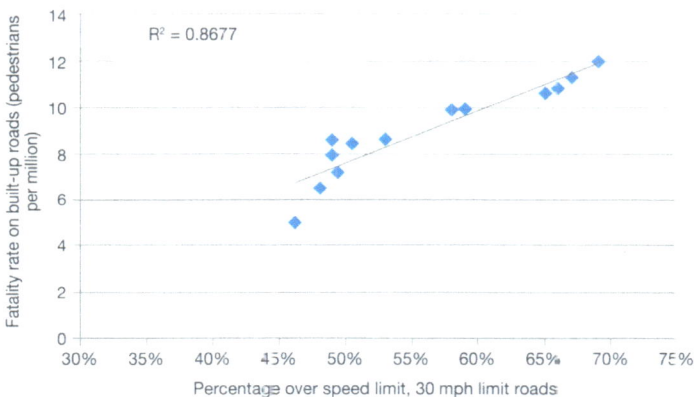

Figure 7.2 Pedestrian fatality rate on built-up roads per million population plotted against the percentage of cars exceeding the 30 mph limit (Source: Mitchell 2012, Fig. 4)

The pedestrian fatality rate on built-up roads per million population against the proportion of cars exceeding the 30 mph limit on built-up roads is based on annual statistics which show good correlation. Figure 7.2 plots the pedestrian fatality rate on built-up roads per million population against the proportion of cars exceeding the 30 mph limit on built-up roads. The resulting scatter plot can be reasonably fitted by a straight line. This means that changes in the percentage of cars exceeding the speed limit is associated with the change in pedestrian fatalities.

However, statistical correlation does not necessarily imply cause; both speed and fatality rate could vary together because of changes in some other factor, with no causal link between them. Other research has identified a link between speed and casualties; for example, multiple Royal Society for the Prevention of Accidents (RoSPA) (2011) studies, summarised in Table 7.1, have shown that pedestrians will be more severely injured, or killed, when hit by cars at higher speeds, and particularly when the car is travelling at more than 30 mph.

A recent analysis of the role of vehicle speed in pedestrian fatalities in Great Britain (DfT 2010), found that 85% of pedestrians killed when struck by cars or car-derived vans died in collisions at impact speeds below 40 mph, 45% at less than 30 mph and 5% at speeds below 20 mph. The risk of a pedestrian being killed when hit by a car increases slowly until impact speeds of around 30 mph. Above this speed, the risk quickly increases, so that a pedestrian being killed by a car travelling at between 30 mph and 40 mph is 3.5 to 5.5 times more likely than if hit by a car travelling below 30 mph. However, about half of pedestrian fatalities occur at impact speeds of 30 mph or below. Elderly pedestrians have a much greater risk of suffering fatal injuries than other age groups.

Country	Date	Number of injuries examined	Risk of fatal injury at 30 mph	Increased risk of fatal injury between 30 and 40 mph
UK	1970s	358	9%	5.5 times more likely
Germany	1999-2007	490 (excludes children under 15)	7%	3.5 times more likely
UK	2000-09	197	7%	4.5 times more likely

Table 7.1 Pedestrian fatality risk (DfT, 2010)

Reducing Speed-related Casualties (Based on RoSPA 2011)

The dangers caused by driving at inappropriate speeds must be clearly explained and demonstrated (in the way that has been done for drink-driving) in order to work towards a general acceptance and ownership of the problem of illegal and inappropriate speed.

Persuading people to drive at safer speeds will be easier if they understand and accept that driving too fast significantly increases the chances of an accident, and significantly increases the chances of that accident being serious or fatal. Road safety publicity campaigns such as the Government's THINK! road safety campaign and the Scottish Government's 'Foolsspeed' campaign are strongly supported by major road safety organisations.

Unfortunately, road safety education and publicity are often undermined in the mass media. Motor manufacturers, and their advertising companies, continue to emphasise the speed and power of their vehicles. Television motoring programmes continue to promote the thrill of speed, placing undue emphasis on performance at speed, often showing cars being raced (albeit not on the public highway). Television dramas often show characters driving too fast when speeding is not essential to the plot or the characterisation.

Motor manufacturers, national press, TV and advertisers should not glamourise speed as exciting and exhilarating nor as 'normal' behaviour. The Advertising Standards Authority (ASA) has taken action on a number of occasions against car advertisements that promote speed, and this is very welcome. The ASA and other broadcast regulatory bodies could usefully review and strengthen their guidance in this respect. RoSPA has produced a guide (2004) to help those working in the media to avoid inadvertently showing potentially dangerous road user behaviour.

Driver Education and Training

Speeding is a symptom of a more general poor attitude towards driving. One of the weaknesses of the UK's driver licensing system is that once the driving test has been passed, the driver is licensed, virtually for life, with no requirement and very little incentive to develop his or her driving abilities or skills further. Drivers can voluntarily take further training, such as Pass Plus or courses offered by driver training providers such as RoSPA, but there is little incentive for individual drivers to do so. Only 3% of drivers take any further driving instruction after passing their test (West 1998). Therefore, there is a need to develop new ways of encouraging drivers to continue to develop their driving skills after the test.

Over the last 15 years or so in Britain, the driver training regime and the driving test have been enhanced. Ways of improving the road environment to encourage drivers to drive at appropriate speeds are discussed in *Helping Drivers Not To Speed* (RoSPA 2007), and advice on how to avoid inadvertently exceeding the speed limit is provided in RoSPA's Top Ten Tips To Stay Within the Limit (RoSPA 2007). Also, a wide range of good practice guidelines have been published by DfT and the Chartered Institution of Highways and Transportation (CIHT).

20 mph Zones

Safer roads benefit all road users, but especially those most vulnerable: pedestrians, cyclists, motorcyclists, children and older people. The most effective measures in reducing vehicle speeds, and thereby decreasing road death and injury, are area-wide traffic calming schemes and 20 mph zones.

20 mph zones are areas where the speed limit has been set at 20 mph and traffic calming measures have been put in place to encourage drivers to stay within this limit. A Transport Research Laboratory

(TRL) review (1996) of accident data in seventy-two 20 mph zones found that average mean speeds were reduced by 9 mph, from 25 mph to 16 mph in the zones. On average, for every 1 mph speed reduction, there was a 6.2% accident reduction. All road accidents in the zones fell by 61%, and there was no evidence of accident migration onto surrounding roads. The effects were particularly significant for the most vulnerable road users in that:

- all pedestrian accidents decreased by 63%;
- child accidents decreased by 67%; and,
- child pedestrian accidents decreased by 70%.

In London, a Transport for London (TfL) review (2003) of over one hundred 20 mph zones in London also found that they were very effective in reducing road injuries to children. In these zones, speeds were reduced by 9 mph and traffic flows by about 15%. Pedestrian casualties were down by 40%, and pedestrians killed or seriously injured (KSI) down by 50%. Child pedestrian casualties decreased by 48% and child pedestrians KSI decreased by 61%.

Enforcement

Deaths and injuries caused by poor, and often illegal, behaviour on the road far exceeds the number of people killed through any other form of crime. A clearly effective way of enforcing speed limits has been shown by the use of safety cameras (also sometimes referred to by some agencies and researchers as 'speed cameras').

An independent review (University College London and PA Consulting 2005) of more than 4,000 safety cameras over a four-year period shows conclusively that cameras significantly reduce speeding and collisions, and cut deaths and serious injuries at camera sites by 42%. This means there were 1,745 fewer people being killed or seriously injured at the camera sites per year – including 100 fewer deaths per year. Regarding pedestrians:

- The number of children killed and seriously injured at camera sites decreased by 32%.
- The number of pedestrians killed or seriously injured fell by 29% at camera sites.

A review of the evidence of the effectiveness of speed cameras in 2010 (Allsop 2010) examined data from UK and international studies along with data on traffic speeds, collisions and casualties. Taking into account other factors that might reduce speed and speed-related crashes and casualties, such as the downward national trend in casualty numbers, the review concluded that in the year ending March 2004, cameras at more than 4,000 sites across Great Britain prevented some 3,600 personal injury collisions, saving around 1,000 people from being killed or seriously injured. The report also concluded that if safety cameras were decommissioned about 800 extra people across Great Britain could be killed or seriously injured each year.

Vehicle Engineering

Motor manufacturers could play a much more prominent role in reducing the number of people killed and injured in speed-related road accidents. Manufacturers continue to produce cars and motorcycles that are capable of achieving speeds of 160 mph and more. RoSPA believes that the European Commission, national governments and the motor industry should work together to develop restrictions on the top speeds and power of new cars and motorcycles.

Modern cars provide a smooth, quiet drive, even at very high speeds, and therefore drivers are often insulated from any real sensation of the speed at which they are travelling. The vehicle's power means that it is very easy to creep above the speed limit. Indeed, drivers often cite this as a reason for speeding.

Intelligent Speed Adaptation

Technology which can prevent drivers from exceeding the speed limit on any particular road is being developed and tested. The latest field tests (University of Leeds and MIRA Ltd 2008) show that this *"is now a mature technology which is capable of delivering substantial reductions in excessive speed and thereby considerable benefits in terms of safety"*.

Intelligent Speed Adaptation (ISA) is a system by which the vehicle 'knows' the permitted or recommended maximum speed for a road. The standard system uses an in-vehicle digital road map onto which speed limits have been coded, combined with a positioning system which could be GPS, i.e. the satellite Global Positioning System, but could also be GPS-enhanced with map matching and dead reckoning.

ISA can take various forms: in terms of intervention level it can be advisory (the driver is informed of the limit and of violations), voluntary (the system is linked to the vehicle controls but the driver can choose when to have the system enabled), or mandatory (no override is possible). The speed limit information can potentially be extended to incorporate lower speeds at certain locations on the road system and even variation within it based on weather, traffic density, incidents etc.

Depending on how the technology is implemented, over the 60-year period from 2010 to 2070, it would be expected to reduce fatal accidents by between 10% (approximately 15,400 fatal accidents) and 26% (approximately 43,300 fatal accidents), serious injury accidents between 6% (96,000 accidents) and 21% (330,000 accidents), and slight injury accidents by between 3% (336,000 accidents) and 12% (1.3 million accidents).

One of the requirements for the widespread implementation of this technology is a digital map showing the speed limit on every road in the country, which can easily and regularly be updated, including taking account of speed limit changes due to road works. Ultimately, this will make it possible to display the speed limit of every road within the car, so that a driver can constantly be aware of the limit.

Some satellite navigation devices can also advise drivers of the speed limit of the road, although drivers should still primarily rely on the legal road signs, in case the device is not up to date or malfunctioning, or if a temporary limit is in place.

Employers

Driving is the most dangerous work activity that most people do (RoSPA 2011). Health and Safety Executive (HSE) guidelines, *Driving at Work* (HSE & DfT 2003), state that "health and safety law applies to on-the-road work activities, as do all work activities, and the risks should be effectively managed within a health and safety system".

Employers should identify high risk drivers and high risk journeys and set schedules that are generous enough to ensure that drivers are not time-pressured into speeding and must comply with posted speed limits when driving.

RoSPA has produced a guide, *Driving for Work: Safer Speed Policy* (RoSPA 2004), to help employers and line managers to ensure that their staff are not tempted or pressurised into driving at inappropriate speeds. It includes a sample 'Safer Speed Policy' which can be adopted as written or adapted to suit an organisation's needs.

ALCOHOL – DRINKING AND DRIVING
(Road safety information August 2013, RoSPA)

In 2011, provisional figures showed that 280 people were killed, 1,290 were seriously injured and there were almost 10,000 casualties in total in drink-drive accidents in the UK (DfT 2012). Although the level of drinking and driving has dropped dramatically over the last three decades, almost 300 people are still killed in drink-drive accidents every year (about 1 in 6 of all road deaths).

Often it is an innocent person who suffers, not the driver who is over the drink-drive limit.

In 2012, as shown in Table 7.2, 10 pedestrians were reported killed, 90 KSI and 290 KSI or slightly injured.

Casualty Category	Number
Fatal	10
Serious injury	80
Slight injury	109
All severities	290

Table 7.2 Estimated reported drink-drive accidents by pedestrian involvement, 2012 (Based on RRCGB 2013, Table RAS50004)

As well as excessive alcohol use of drivers, pedestrians too can become casualties due to drunkenness. Berrymans Lace Mawer (2008) states: "The problem is that in their drunken state they probably think that they are invulnerable and take little heed of normal road safety precautions. Unfortunately for the driver, they are just one more hazard to be aware of, perhaps regarding them in the same light as young children. Furthermore, the courts seem unwilling to place all the blame on the pedestrian, even in cases of extreme drunkenness."

Lower Drink-Drive Limit

RoSPA (2015) believes that the maximum blood alcohol limit in the UK should be lowered from 80 mg of alcohol per 100 ml of blood

(80 mg/100 ml) to 50 mg of alcohol per 100 ml of blood (50 mg/100 ml). The current limit was based on evidence that the likelihood of a road accident rises sharply at and above that level. The evidence also showed that most drivers are impaired and their risk increases below this limit. However, in Scotland in 2014 the alcohol limit for drivers was reduced to 50 mg of alcohol in every 100 ml of blood. The Scottish Government says it has changed its drink-drive limit to bring Scotland in line with most other European countries, to save lives and make Scotland's roads safer. In most other European countries, the limit is usually 50 mg per 100 ml of blood.

In 2010, the then Government commissioned Sir Peter North to conduct the North Review of Drink and Drug Driving Law (North 2010). Evidence was given to the Review (RoSPA 2010) and calls for a lower limit were made based on evidence that drivers with a blood alcohol level of between 50 mg and 80 mg are 2–2.5 times more likely to be involved in an accident than drivers without alcohol, and up to six times more likely to be in a fatal crash (Department of the Environment, Transport and the Regions (DETR) 1998).

The North Review *estimated that the impact of any lowering in the blood alcohol limit will reduce casualties following implementation, with an estimate of up to 303 lives annually saved by the sixth year. The report recommended that* the limit be lowered to 50 mg of alcohol per 100 ml of blood. The estimates do not include Scotland, which accounts for about 7% of drink-drive-related casualties in Great Britain, so the overall number of lives saved would be even greater.

In 2011 the British Government decided not to lower the limit as it concluded that improving enforcement is likely to have more impact on the most dangerous drink-drivers than lowering the drink-drive limit itself, which it did not believe would be cost-effective (DfT 2011).

Both Scotland and Northern Ireland propose similar limits and RoSPA supports the Scottish and Northern Ireland proposals to lower the drink-drive limit but also believes that it should be lowered across the whole of the UK. Other matters under consideration include lower legal limits for young drivers; breath testing (random, without prior suspicion, evidential roadside); and enforcement levels.

In its response (Centre for Public Health Excellence, *NICE* 2010) to the North Report, the Government announced it would implement a number of measures, which RoSPA supports, to improve the enforcement process. These include:

- Revoking the right people have to opt for a blood test when their evidential breath test result is less than 40% over the limit (sometimes the delay in obtaining a blood test means that the alcohol in a driver's body has fallen below the limit even though they were above the limit when they took the roadside breath test, and so some drivers who had been drinking and driving 'get away with it').
- Streamlining the procedure for testing drink-drivers in hospital.
- Closing a loophole used by high-risk offenders to delay their medical examinations (sometimes the loophole has allowed them to regain their licence at the end of their disqualification period before they have taken and passed the mandatory medical examination that high-risk offenders are required to take).
- Requiring serious drink-drivers to take remedial training and a linked driving assessment – as well as a medical examination – before recovering their licence.
- Relaunching the drink-drive rehabilitation scheme under which drink-drivers can obtain reduced driving disqualifications.
- Approving portable evidential breath-testing equipment for the police.
- Providing for preliminary testing not to be required where evidential testing can be undertaken away from the police station (this will allow evidential breath tests to be conducted at the roadside using portable breath testing equipment mentioned above).

Penalties and Deterrents

Measures under consideration (RoSPA 2015) include:

- **Disqualification periods**. A further measure would be to ensure that where an offender is imprisoned as well as disqualified from driving, the disqualification period does not begin until they have been released from prison.
- **Immediate licence confiscation for failing a breath test.** This would be effective but difficult to enforce; since drivers do not have to carry a licence in this country, it is difficult to see how this could be enforced.
- **Seizing vehicles of repeat drink-drive offenders.** This would be a significant deterrent to drink-driving.
- **High Risk Offenders' Scheme**. Offenders should be required to take an extended driving test at the end of their disqualification before being able to regain their driving licence.
- **Drink-drive courses**. Wider use of sanctions designed to change offenders' behaviour, such as rehabilitation courses and retesting, could be beneficial. In November 2011 the Driving Standards Agency (DSA) published a consultation paper (DSA 2011) on proposals to improve drink-drive rehabilitation courses and to encourage more training providers to become involved in giving the courses.
- **Alcohol ignition interlock devices (Alcolocks)**. Designed to prevent a car engine from starting if the person who breathes into the device has been drinking alcohol. There is some evidence that they are effective in discouraging reoffending while the order is in force, but that reoffending occurs once the restriction is removed. The main problems reported by participants included being over the interlock limit the morning after drinking, delay in starting the car due to the time taken for the interlock to warm up and difficulties with rolling retests during a journey. Many of the participants indicated that the devices made them at least think seriously about their drinking, if not help change their drinking patterns outright.

[Author's note: There is no technical reason why vehicles cannot be fitted with a breathaliser which would prevent the vehicle from starting if the level of alcohol detected were over a certain limit. This device could be so designed and located that it would render the vehicle unstartable if tampered with. Penalties for professional disabling of the device could be severe. A vehicle driven by a driver who is 'over the limit' is as lethal as a loaded firearm in the hands of a drunk. Action is needed to limit the damage such a combination can cause.]

- **Education and publicity**. Publicity and education campaigns conducted since the late 1970s have changed public knowledge and attitudes about drinking and driving. Long-term publicity is essential, supported by education programmes for school children and drivers. Given the very large proportion of the population in this category this will mean a major change in the nation's drinking habits with related health benefits which in turn should be included in any overall cost-benefit analysis.
- **Alcohol unit labelling**. The drinks industry could give clearer advice on alcohol content on labels and at point of sale. Research is needed on the best way to convey the message on alcohol content.
- **Alternatives to drinking and driving**. The drinks industry should adopt a more enthusiastic marketing approach to promote a positive image for low-alcohol or alcohol-free drinks and introduce a price advantage for these drinks.
- **Self-test breathalysers**. Many different types of self-test breathalysers are available, ranging from very cheap 'blow-in-a-bag' devices to more expensive digital models. They tend to be marketed as a means for drivers to check whether they are over the limit, particularly the morning after they have been drinking. RoSPA is concerned that self-test breathalysers may be inaccurate and may encourage people to try to drink up to the limit and drive, rather than plan ahead, and if they are intending to drink alcohol to make arrangements (taxis, designated drivers, etc.) so that they do not need to drive. There might be a useful 'morning after' role for self-test breathalysers, but only if their

accuracy could be relied upon and people understand how to use them properly and do not misuse them.

DRIVER INEXPERIENCE – YOUNG DRIVERS

The high incidence of accidents caused by inexperienced drivers is of considerable concern, and organisations such as BRAKE (2015) and RoSPA (2015) have addressed key issues. As well as matters affecting the general public, the insurance industry has an interest in this area, both in terms of pressures to reduce insurance premiums and its role in promoting public safety. A recent presentation (Pendry 2014) summarised many of the issues, including calls to implement Graduated Driver Licensing (GDL). The remainder of this chapter summarises the main features of this speech.

With young drivers grossly overrepresented in the insurance industry's claim statistics, there is particular interest in improving young drivers' road safety record. The most recent data shows that:

- nearly a quarter of all car drivers who died in 2012 were young drivers – this is despite the fact people aged between 17 and 24 make up only around 8% of all driving licence holders in Great Britain;
- 40% of 17-year-old men have a crash in their first six months of driving.

The reality is that the biggest single cause of accidental death amongst young people is getting in a car and dying in a crash.

The insurance industry has always approached the young driver problem from a road safety perspective, not a financial one. The key outcome we should all be aiming for is to improve the safety of young drivers by improving the way they learn to drive. That their insurance premiums will reduce as a result should be a secondary consideration. However, motor insurance is a compulsory purchase.

It is recognised that the ability of young people to drive is key to their social and economic participation in society. And in difficult economic times, relatively high premiums for young drivers are a cause of real concern.

The insurance industry supports any measures that are proven – really proven – to improve the road safety of young drivers, and believes that the single most effective measure the UK could adopt is the introduction of GDL. This method is a way of allowing new drivers to build driving experience under low-risk conditions. A minimum learning period of one year, followed by a short period of restrictions, will provide young drivers with strong encouragement to obtain plenty of practical experience. A six-month period of restrictions would follow.

Firstly, the newly qualified driver is unable to drive with passengers under the age of 21 who are not immediate family because the presence of young passengers in a car can both distract young drivers and encourage them to drive in a more risky way.

Secondly, the night-time restriction is because numerous studies have clearly demonstrated that driving during the night increases the crash risk among young drivers for a variety of reasons including driver fatigue, lack of sustained night-time driving experience and recreational driving at night.

Lifting these restrictions after six months will ensure young drivers have built up the skills and experience required to drive on their own. Exemptions will apply to the restrictions, such as if a young person needs to go to night-time study or employment.

The international evidence that GDL works is overwhelming and the recent Transport Research Laboratory study into GDL – which was commissioned by DfT – is unequivocal in its support for it, concluding that the case for introducing graduated licensing in the UK is compelling.

In addition to GDL the role that telematics-based products can play shows real promise. These policies use technology to monitor driver behaviour, often adjusting premiums or providing other incentives based on that feedback. And pay-how-you-drive policies offer young people more choice in the insurance products they can purchase. For those young drivers who opt to have their driving behaviour monitored, the technology has been proven to reduce the cost of their car insurance.

However, to what extent it changes the attitude of all road users – as opposed to those drivers who self-select into using the technology – remains to be evaluated, and a government review of the evidence is encouraging.

But, given the current low take-up of telematics, and the time needed to put together a robust research project and to carry out an effective analysis, it is not inconceivable to suggest that DfT is calling for research that could take up to 10 years to produce an answer.

Set against the fact that GDL is here, right now, and works, it is very disappointing that its introduction is not being considered. GDL is based on sound evidence and to ignore that evidence by failing to act is resulting in catastrophic results for many young drivers and high premiums for far too many. Evidence is important as almost every week the industry is asked by various road safety initiatives if their members would reduce their insurance premiums for individuals who have attended some form of road safety course.

The idea that the key to improving young driver safety is to provide them with better education remains pervasive. But unfortunately the only direct benefit imparted by such education is basic vehicle control skills and knowledge of the rules of the road. *According to the evidence, education alone has no measurable direct effect on young driver collision risk and, therefore, its continued use should be set against much lower expectations in terms of what it can contribute to road safety compared to GDL.*

Likewise, the assumption that vehicle-handling skills are deficient among drivers contributes to the widespread availability of programmes such as under-17 car park courses that train young drivers how to handle vehicles in advanced driving situations. These courses may actually give young drivers a false sense of their abilities, leading them to feel overconfident and therefore presenting an even greater danger on the road.

Ultimately, our highly permissive driver training and testing regime has catastrophic results for a few and expensive premiums for far too many.

★

> The involvement of speeding, use of alcohol and driving by inexperienced, primarily young, drivers in road casualties, and their particularly severe effects on pedestrians and other vulnerable road users present a continuing challenge. Regarding speeding, greater awareness of the beneficial effects of implementing selected 20 mph speed limits is increasingly realised, and enforcement, driver education and training, vehicle engineering and employers' involvement can all play their part. Concerning alcohol, as illustrated by the recent actions of the Scottish Government, it is evident that legislation to reduce levels of alcohol in drivers is feasible and measures ranging from disqualification to self-test breathalysers and alcohol ignition interlock systems could receive greater emphasis. Measures to address deaths and injuries resulting from inexperienced drivers would benefit from implementation of GDL (but keeping awareness of the ineffectiveness of advanced training for this group) with accompanying advantages to young drivers, pedestrians and other road users.

References – Speed

Allsop, R. (November 2010) *The Effectiveness of Speed Cameras: A Review of Evidence*. RAC Foundation, London.

Department for Transport (September 2010) *Relationship between Speed and Risk of Fatal Injury: Pedestrians and Car Occupants*, Road Safety Web Publication No.16. London.

Department for Transport (2011) Reported Road Casualties Great Britain (RRCGB) *2010 Contributory Factors to Reported Road Accidents*. London.

Health and Safety Executive and Department for Transport (2003) *Driving at Work: Managing Work Related Road Safety* INDG 382. London.

http://assets.dft.gov.uk/statistics/releases/road-accidents-and-safety-annual-report-2010/rrcgb2010-04.pdf

Mitchell, C.G.B. (2012) *Speed and Safety. Evidence from Published Data*. RAC Foundation, London.

Royal Society for the Prevention of Accidents (2004) *Driving for Work: Safer Speed Policy*. London.

Royal Society for the Prevention of Accidents (2004) *Presenting Road Safety: A Guide for the Media*. London.

Royal Society for the Prevention of Accidents (2007) *Helping Drivers Not To Speed*. London.

Royal Society for the Prevention of Accidents (2007) *Top Ten Tips to Stay Within the Limit*. London.

Royal Society for the Prevention of Accidents (2011) Inappropriate *Speed*. London.

Royal Society for the Prevention of Accidents (2015) *Road Safety Information*. London.

Transport Research Laboratory (1996) Report No. 215 *Review of Traffic Calming Schemes in 20 mph Zones*. Crowthorne.

Transport for London (2003) *Review of 20 mph Zones in London Boroughs. TfL Safety Research Report*, London.

University College London & PA Consulting (2005) *The National Safety Camera Programme: Four-year Evaluation Report*. London.

University of Leeds and MIRA Ltd (June 2008) *Isa-UK Intelligent Speed Adaptation: Final Report*. Leeds.

West, R. (1998) *Accident Rates and Behavioural Characteristics of Novice Drivers in the TRL Cohort Study*, TRL Report 293. Crowthorne.

References – Alcohol

Berrymans Lace Mawer (2008) *Pedestrian Claims*. Motor Claims Update_MGB, PNG, PEN_(RAW, ACH) 11/08.

Centre for Public Health Excellence/National Institute for Health and Care Excellence (2010) *Review of effectiveness of laws limiting blood alcohol concentration levels to reduce alcohol-related road injuries and deaths*. London.

Department for Transport (March 2011) *The Government's Response to the Reports by Sir Peter North CBE QC and the Transport Select Committee on Drink and Drug Driving Law*. London

Department for Transport (2012) *Reported Road Casualties in Great Britain: 2011 Provisional Estimates for Accidents Involving Illegal Alcohol Levels*. London.

Department for Transport (August 2012) www.dft.gov.uk/statistics/releases/road-accidents-and-safety-drink-drive-estimates-2011.

Department of the Environment, Transport and the Regions (1998) *Combating Drink Driving: Next Steps: A Consultation Paper.* London.

Driving Standards Agency (November 2011) *New Approval Arrangements for Drink Drive Rehabilitation Courses: A Consultation Paper.* London

North, Sir P. (June 2010) *Report of the Review of Drink and Drug Driving Law.* London.

Royal Society for the Prevention of Accidents (February 2010) *RoSPA's Submission to the North Review of Drink and Drug Driving Law.* London.

Royal Society for the Prevention of Accidents (2015) *Drink Driving* website. London.

www.rospa.com/roadsafety/consultations/2010/north_review_written_submission.pdf

References – Driver Inexperience

BRAKE (2015) *Young Drivers*. Website accessed June 2015.

Pendry, S. (2014) *The insurance industry and road safety: current and future policy priorities.* Speech at Inside Government forum on the Future of Road Safety in the UK. London.

Royal Society for the Prevention of Accidents (2015) *Young Drivers*. London.

CHAPTER 8

EVENT DATA RECORDING – THE BLACK BOX

Can information improve performance?

Documenting events in an unbiased, transparent way can assist in investigating the circumstances of those events. This lack of bias can, with sensitive interpretation, enable informed analysis for examining reasons for an 'accident' and enable investigation of how, when and where it happened. It also has been shown that if a person's actions are recorded and therefore will be available for future scrutiny, greater care will be taken in conducting such action. The application to in-vehicle recording of events is therefore clear. Yet, for pedestrians, further research is needed in recording responsiveness to collisions with such 'soft' objects – accidents which typically involve minimal reduction in velocity of a vehicle but which can be lethal to a pedestrian. Despite its considerable potential, acceptance of the event data recorders (EDRs) by drivers will be a considerable challenge.

★

Description and Installation

Known generally as an event data recorder (EDR), installed in a vehicle it "… works by constantly monitoring vehicle acceleration and deceleration – key features of a suddenly occurring event – as well as other features such as seat belt use, braking, swerving etc. These inputs are stored for a few seconds until overwritten with new data. This creates a window of data typically 5 sec long that is constantly being overwritten. If the acceleration exceeds a certain trigger level, normally about 2g, as would occur in a collision, the

EDR stores all the preceding data permanently. This can then be downloaded and analysed to assist in understanding how a collision occurs." (Safety Rating Advisory Committee (SARAC) II 2005 a)

The exact operation of a particular EDR will depend on the manufacturer's model and requirements: recording times vary, video and audio may also be included, different 'trigger' levels at which specific items of information are recorded may be used as well as differences in the inputs.

Modern EDRs are about the size of a cigarette packet, but this may vary depending on the type and number of inputs. Generally located under a passenger seat where they are protected from collision damage, they record approximately the same acceleration movement (such movements may occur in any direction, including reverse, sideways or vertically, which may be experienced in a crash) or 'pulse' as is experienced by the vehicle occupants.

An estimated 65-90% of all 2004 model year cars were fitted with some kind of EDR device in the USA, with more than half being able to record the pulse which occurs in a crash (National Highway Traffic Safety Administration (NHTSA) 2004). A mass produced model may cost less that $100. An example of an EDR is shown in Figure 8.1 and its typical location in a vehicle is shown in Figure 8.2.

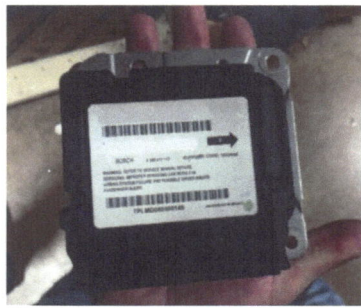

Figure 8.1 An event data recorder (Source: United States Congressional Research Service 2014)

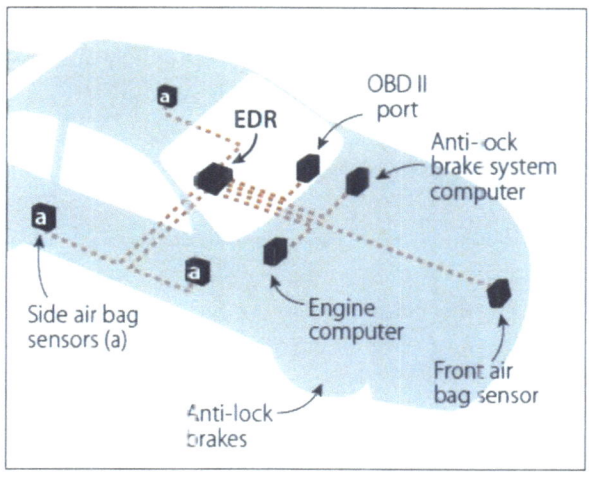

Figure 8.2 The EDR system in a motor vehicle (Source: United States Congressional Research Service 2014)

Insurance companies in particular can benefit from the use of EDRs. For example, they can install the device free of charge and list the following advantages:
- The time of day or night you drive
- The speed you drive at on different sorts of road
- If you brake or accelerate sharply
- If you take breaks on long journeys
- Your motorway miles
- Your total mileage
- The total number of journeys you make

EDR Capabilities

Further developments of EDRs (SARAC 2004 b) include a near miss and accident driver recorder (NADR), which records both accident and near miss data, devised by a Japanese research group. A near miss includes rapid braking, acceleration and steering operations without resulting in a collision. The NADR also measures pitch and roll of the vehicle. An attached video recording assists accuracy in accident analysis, particularly if pedestrians or cyclists are involved, and possible monitoring of driver behaviour.

As well as the EDR, various closely related features are available, including journey data recording (JDR), which shows how a vehicle is being driven at 1-sec intervals. This is useful for instruction and driver monitoring, but detail is usually insufficient for accident analysis. Other terms include sensing and diagnostic modules (SDM), accident data recorder (ADR) and incident data recorder (IDR).

Benefits of EDRs include resolution of insurance claims, accident behaviour and research. More specific focus can be directed at attention deficit and performance research, driver drowsiness and inattention to forward roadway conditions. Knowledge and information in these areas can then assist in combatting attention deficits by means of regular training, monitoring as part of data management, providing driver feedback and periodic vehicle testing.

A particular development reported in one study describes driver monitoring by means of the DRIVE CAM which records red light running, falling asleep and drowsiness, and can thereby assist in retraining and potential legal proceedings. An accident reduction of up to 62% is claimed (DriveCam 2004).

Installation of EDR devices can be more effectively achieved within commercial or institutional groups, often with vehicle fleet ownership or involvement. For this reason, target groups for implementing EDR include:

- commercial organisations operating vehicles such as vans, buses, coaches, heavy goods vehicles;
- motorcyclists;
- young drivers (drivers under the age of 23 cause 25% of all car accidents with personal injuries; EDR should become mandatory for them);

- public authority vehicles, as 'best practice' examples;
- private cars of firefighters – accidents occurring when firefighters respond to the fire department in case of emergency (many accidents occur when firefighters are travelling to the event);
- driver training agencies – enhancements result from training, tuition, vehicle and infrastructure redesign;
- public road maintenance agencies – events resulting from poor maintenance may be recorded by EDR; and,
- elderly drivers.

Driver Behaviour

"In Great Britain, the Netherlands, and Belgium nine vehicle fleets with a total of 443 vehicles fitted with data recording equipment participated in the research Program SAMOVAR conducted within the EU DRIVE Project V 2007. Together with a control panel involved in similar tests a total of 850 vehicles participated. The data, collected over 12 months, showed that the crash rate decreased by 28.1% by use of the vehicle data recorder. The SAMOVAR report finally concluded that the intelligent use of a vehicle data recorder is able to make a considerable, distinctive and independent benefit to road safety." (SARAC 2004 c). Key findings indicate that:

- people who know they are being observed alter their behaviour;
- EDRs reduce collisions when drivers are aware the recorders have been fitted;
- there has been a 28.1% reduction in the monthly accident rate per vehicle in vehicles with EDRs;
- EDR data gives faster analysis than does conventional crash investigation;
- there has been a 20% reduction in collisions in Berlin police radio patrol vehicles – all vehicles are now fitted with EDRs; and,
- there has been a 20% reduction in crashes in car, truck and coach fleets.

Further evidence of potential benefits of EDR (Vehicle Event Recording Based on Intelligent Crash Assessment (VERONICA II a 2009)) indicates that in parallel with the use of EDR as an enforcement device, the most important direct effect of EDR in terms of road security concerns driver behaviour: drivers can be expected to modify their behaviour accordingly knowing that traffic law infringements can, in principle, be detected if an 'accident-event' should occur.

A cost-benefit assessment and prioritisation study of 21 vehicle safety technologies conducted for the European Commission in 2005, and based on a wide range of EDR field examples and studies, concludes an average reduction of collision probability of 10% for fatalities as well as for serious and light injuries (VERONICA II a 2009). Benefits are estimated to outweigh costs by a factor of 7.

EDR can also assist victims of a crash who are unable to summon help; in receiving prompt notification of the time and place of an accident emergency services can be immediately dispatched to a location recorded by the Global Positioning System (GPS) incorporated in the EDR. Initial results have been obtained using the E-call system contact with public safety answering point (PSAP), which, however, is still under development.

Studies (VERONICA II b 2009) show that 5.4% of injured people are unable to contact rescue services in urban areas – 11.8% in rural areas – and that attention to crash victims is extremely beneficial if conducted within the 'golden hour' when medical assistance is often crucial to a victim's survival. Considerably more work needs to be done, however, to ensure that this system is effective.

The 'Trigger' Issue

A continuing issue in the uses of EDR in collisions with vulnerable road users is the matter of the 'trigger' conditions which start a recording on the EDR (SARAC 2004).

As described (VERONICA II c 2009), 'triggering' means to start the recording (freezing) of data continuously generated, once a certain accident severity (i.e. the 'trigger' threshold) is reached. If the threshold is not reached data are continuously overwritten by new data, i.e. they are neither stored nor recorded.

Collisions with vulnerable road users are considered to require a threshold defined as a change in vehicle velocity that equals or exceeds 8 km/h within a 0.15 sec interval. This change in velocity event definition is not sufficient to record all relevant accidents, e.g. cars with two-wheelers or with pedestrians (vulnerable road users), or heavy goods vehicles (HGVs) with cars. Research in the USA reveals that present trigger technology leaves many events with low changes in velocity without airbag deployment, i.e. unrecorded, and others with high uncertainties.

Trigger requirements in the light of the (VERONICA II d 2009) mission indicate that intelligent combinations of several, but not necessarily complicated, trigger parameters are necessary. Based on almost 3,000 real-life accident experiences it was found that 93% of all accidents come to a standstill within 3 sec following the first impact. Regarding technical feasibility, therefore, triggering could not only rely on the change in velocity but also on deployable devices such as pop-up bonnets and external airbags, or by camera, radar or other technical means.

Collisions known as 'soft object' also include those involving trucks and passenger vehicles which occur typically with low changes in velocity when the impact occurs and are therefore difficult to distinguish from hard braking (VERONICA II e 2009). A solution would be to record all collisions. However, storage capacity restrictions and data privacy concerns prevent this. Therefore, a more intelligent trigger has to be considered, that may be called a 'corrected trigger', when the change in velocity is equal to or greater than 2 km/h within 0.12 sec.

An Example of a 'Soft Object' Trigger

A pedestrian crossing from the left crashed with her head into the windscreen of a bus, and was fatally injured (VERONICA II f, 2009). Police suspected that the bus's right indicator had been set to stop at a bus stop, thus misleading the pedestrian into thinking that it was safe to cross the street. This was rebutted by an automatic data recording (ADR) triggered automatically and by a standstill trigger. The NHTSA standard trigger would not have recorded the crash (soft object and no airbag in the bus anyway). Figure 8.3 shows the crash impact location on the bus.

In conclusion, if EDR data is to be used to comprehensively enhance road safety the event definition also has to include the detection of the so-called 'soft object' collisions, i.e. collisions with vulnerable road users. Their share among road victims is considerable. In order that EDRs can record such collisions a trigger specification is required which goes beyond the air-bag-related NHTSA specifications, as these only focus on the protection of the vehicle occupants and not on road users outside the vehicle.

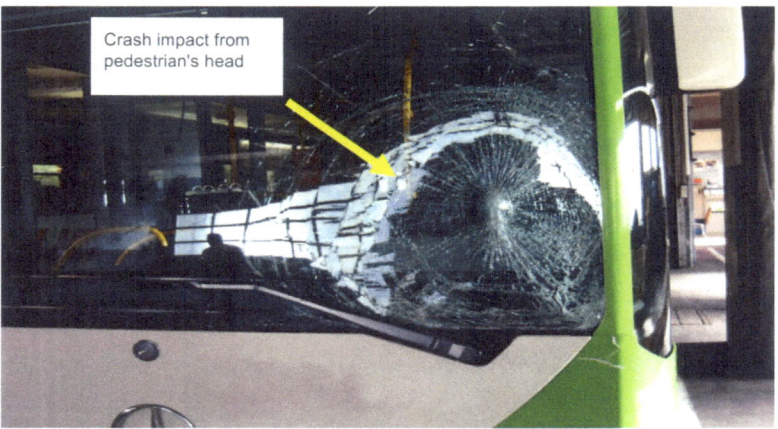

Figure 8.3 Crash impact from pedestrian's head on a bus windscreen

These recommendations were not unanimously agreed upon. Ford Motor Company provided the following comment: "In theory we do not object to including vulnerable road users in the specification of EDRs but we have expressed doubts about the feasibility of doing so, especially in terms of sensor capability and memory capacity. We believe that the greatest benefits can be gained by widespread deployment of EDRs based on technology already available on vehicles but which is not currently capable of robustly recording impacts with low changes in velocity."

Other project partners argued that including collisions with vulnerable road users in the scope of European EDRs might increase the demands placed on vehicle manufacturers in meeting these requirements. However, there is evidence that these requirements can be useful in the detection of collisions with 'soft objects'. Figure 8.4, for example, shows an example of a Dutch ambulance which was involved in a collision with a pedestrian. The vehicle's Airbag Sensing & Diagnostic Module (SDM) 'triggered' the recording of a soft object collision under conditions which the NHTSA standard does not require.

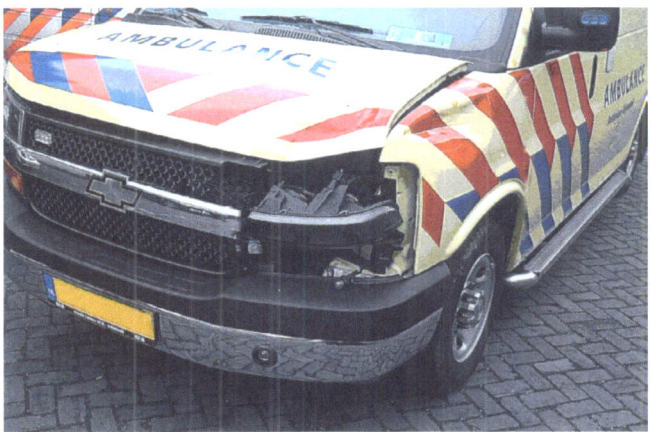

Figure 8.4 Impact damage from a collision between an ambulance and a pedestrian

Despite the fact that trigger events may be difficult to define in terms of impacts with pedestrians, the EDR may still provide useful information in the result of a collision. For example, most drivers when a collision occurs will brake or steer in a direction different from their original path. In the event of a 'hit and run' accident evidence may be available to police through the recording of these events, as well as the time of the accident, which can assist in resolving details of the collision and therefore assigning responsibility.

Administration and Use of EDR Data

The actions and interests of the stakeholders and the flow of information which responds to legal, contractual or business concerns can be divided into groups of public or private interests. Public interests include road transport and traffic enforcement authorities, tribunals and courts, and policy makers and regulators with national and regional interests, police, courts and researchers. Private interests include drivers and vehicle owners, lawyers, insurance companies and third parties such as accident victims, vehicle workshops, manufacturers, and transport lease, rental and fleet interests.

The administrative data flow (ADF) starts, as shown in Figure 8.5 (VERONICA II g 2009), when 'frozen' data is downloaded either by the police, collision experts or vehicle workshops. Within the EDR data framework, law enforcement authorities, including police forces at national and local levels, are the first agencies to intervene, thus initiating or not the investigation of the ADF or EDR data. As police have the obligation to maintain public security and to investigate civil and criminal actions this also includes accidents and crimes related to road safety.

Collision experts might represent either private or public interests. They are often the first stakeholders to handle EDR data as their expertise routinely requires its careful assessment and interpretation.

The services of accident reconstruction experts are generally requested by the prosecutor or the police following an accident.

During the data collection process, it is worthwhile considering that under specific circumstances, EDR data could be downloaded by workshops, or data could be simply collected within a workshop by the police or reconstruction experts. In such a case, workshops would be acting either on behalf of a public authority or, at minimum, under its supervision. Workshops could also extract EDR data upon request of the car owners and drivers. Considering the various threats and challenges to EDR data integrity, workshops could only extract EDR data if given legal authority to do so.

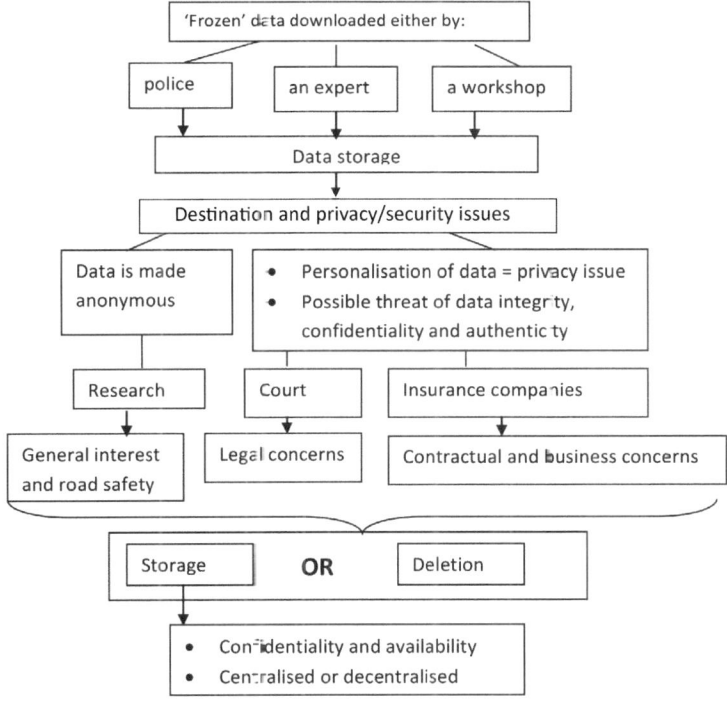

Figure 8.5 Potential administrative data flow (Source: VERONICA II g, Fig. 20 Potential administrative data flow, p. 45)

Practical Issues

The installation and use of 'black boxes' in vehicles is addressed by RoSPA (2013). As well as reporting a wide range of safety benefits and accident reduction with the use of EDRs, the report lists:

> … a reduction rate of 38% in accidents and in unsafe driving practices of 82%; savings in personal and vehicle fleet costs; and potential for improving road safety engineering and research. Attention is drawn to the practicalities of implementation. These include:
>
> - the socio-economic implications of the cost for EDR installation and use;
> - relative advantages and disadvantages of using mobile devices as the EDR unit, having regards to its possible malfunction;
> - how best to channel useful feedback to people responsible for the conduct of drivers in several settings;
> - privacy issues resulting from the availability of data; and,
> - standardisation of equipment, methods and reporting to insurance and telematics companies.

RoSPA (2013) concludes that, "it [EDR] has great potential to significantly improve driving standards and reduce crash and casualty rates. Largely restricted to two groups, young novice drivers and at-work drivers, but could also be used with other groups of drivers, and perhaps eventually be standard technology in all vehicles."

★

To the extent that documented reduction in collisions includes a proportion of pedestrian involvement, EDR has progressed in its application and has shown, especially in commercial and public service vehicle fleets, and for inexperienced, mostly young, drivers, that significant improvements result from its installation. In terms of accident reconstruction, although doubts about the triggering velocity need further examination, the ability of EDR to record the exact time, location, velocity and braking characteristics (except in the case of some 'hit and run' accidents) will assist considerably in determining many of the key events leading to the collision; in combination with camera/video recording it can be valuable in providing forensic, engineering and research analysis improvements. But its greatest benefit is undoubtedly better driving, thereby avoiding accidents in the first place. Regarding its future installation and use generally, the practicalities of installation and using EDR outlined by RoSPA, including possibly mostly privacy issues, will need to be resolved. Nevertheless improvement in driver performance established so far indicates considerable potential benefits for all road users, including pedestrians.

References

Canis, B. and Peterman, D.R. (2014) *"Black Boxes" in Passenger Vehicles: Policy Issues*. Congressional Research Service, Washington DC.

DriveCam (2004) *Event Data Recorders, Vehicle MVideo Recording Systems and Vehicle Monitoring Devices*. Website accessed 2015.

National Highway Traffic Safety Administration/Institute of Electrical and Electronics Engineers (2008 a) Discussion p. 1616, *trigger threshold standard* (Event Data Recorders, Final Rule, 14-01-2008, F.R./Vol.73, p. 2181). Washington DC.

National Highway Traffic Safety Administration/Institute of Electrical and Electronics Engineers (2008 b) Discussion p. 1616, *trigger threshold standard* (Event Data Recorders, Final Rule, 14-01-2008, F.R./Vol.73, p. 2181). Washington DC.

National Highway Traffic Safety Administration (2004) Docket No. NHTSA-2004-18029 Event Data Recorders, Proposal of Rulemaking. Washington DC.

Royal Society for the Prevention of Accidents (2013) *Road Safety and In-Vehicle Monitoring (Black Box) Technology*, Policy Paper. London.

Safety Rating Advisory Committee II a (2005) *Quality Criteria for the Safety Assessment of Cars Based on Real-World Crashes: Scaling Measurement and Improvement of Data Collection, Report of Sub-Task* 1.3/4.3, p. 5.

Safety Rating Advisory Committee II b (2005) *Quality Criteria for the Safety Assessment of Cars Based on Real-World Crashes: Scaling Measurement and Improvement of Data Collection, Report of Sub-Task 1.3/4.3*, p. 14.

Safety Rating Advisory Committee II c (2005) *Quality Criteria for the Safety Assessment of Cars Based on Real-World Crashes: Scaling Measurement and Improvement of Data Collection, Report of Sub-Task 1.3/4.3*, p. 19.

VERONICA II (2009 a) *Vehicle Event Recording Based on Intelligent Crash Assessment*. Final report. European Commission Directorate-General for Energy and Transport. EC Contract No. TREN-07-ST-S07.7-764, p. 39.

VERONICA II (2009 b) *Vehicle Event Recording Based on Intelligent Crash Assessment*. Final report. European Commission Directorate-

General for Energy and Transport. EC Contract No. TREN-07-ST-S07.7-764, p. 20.

VERONICA II (2009 c) *Vehicle Event Recording Based on Intelligent Crash Assessment.* Final report. European Commission Directorate-General for Energy and Transport. EC Contract No. TREN-07-ST-S07.7-764, p. 26.

VERONICA II (2009 d) *Vehicle Event Recording Based on Intelligent Crash Assessment.* Final report. European Commission Directorate-General for Energy and Transport. EC Contract No. TREN-07-ST-S07.7-764, p. 28.

VERONICA II (2009 e) *Vehicle Event Recording Based on Intelligent Crash Assessment.* Final report. European Commission Directorate-General for Energy and Transport. EC Contract No. TREN-07-ST-S07.7-764, p. 29.

VERONICA II (2009 f) *Vehicle Event Recording Based on Intelligent Crash Assessment.* Final report. European Commission Directorate-General for Energy and Transport. EC Contract No. TREN-07-ST-S07.7-764, p. 34.

VERONICA II (2009 g) *Vehicle Event Recording Based on Intelligent Crash Assessment.* Final report. European Commission Directorate-General for Energy and Transport. EC Contract No. TREN-07-ST-S07.7-764, p. 45.

CHAPTER 9

AUTONOMOUS EMERGENCY BRAKING

Avoiding and mitigating collisions

A preferred means of avoiding collision is one in which that most unpredictable element in any crash – the human – is assisted in his or her decision-making and action by a responsive mechanism. Such a technology, known as the Autonomous Emergency Braking (AEB) system, is mostly applicable to avoidance between vehicles. However, it also shows potential for reducing the number and severity of vehicle/pedestrian collisions. This system incorporates forward-looking sensors and/or a camera on a vehicle to identify pedestrians, cyclists and other vulnerable road users as the vehicle approaches them. It can thereby assist the driver or intervene on its own to initiate avoiding action before a collision occurs. A further development is the 'driverless' vehicle, and the implications of this for reducing pedestrian casualties are significant.

Preface to this chapter

Such is the pace of development of so-called 'driverless' cars, the bulk of this chapter concentrates on published research and reports from technical and scientific sources. A postscript addresses more recent, very promising but as yet (January 2017) less reliably verifiable accounts of 'driverless' car developments and potential.

★

Principles of Collision Avoidance

Avoiding or mitigating the severity of collisions between vehicles and pedestrians by means of an early warning to drivers of a critical situation, and/or automatic application of the brakes, will reduce the speed at impact and, therefore, reduce its severity. If detection of obstacles and application of the brakes occur soon enough, the vehicle will stop, thereby avoiding a collision altogether. Limitations include reduced effectiveness at higher vehicle speeds and under lower visibility, drivers' over-reliance on the system to avoid collisions, and legal implications of responsibility in the event of collision.

The presence of AEB means that in instances where the driver does not respond to a warning, emergency braking can still occur as it will only intervene where collisions are deemed imminent and the driver fails to respond.

In studies involving pedestrian/vehicle collisions Rosen et al. (2010) found that the largest benefit of the AEB system was not when the driver had already braked but from occasions when the driver failed to do so. Nearly 80% of the fatality reduction resulted from instances when the driver did not brake and the AEB system had intervened. The remaining contribution came mainly from earlier activation of the brakes by the system where the driver had braked only shortly before impact. The average braking time of drivers who braked was 0.67 sec, whereas the AEB system did so for 1.4 sec. This much longer time when milliseconds are crucial is therefore more effective in reducing the vehicle's speed before an impact and, hence, the severity of injury. Potential collision speed reduction with AEB for drivers having different levels of experience (Ward 2014) are illustrated in Figure 9.1(a) and an example of a driver's view when approaching a pedestrian is shown in Figure 9.1(b).

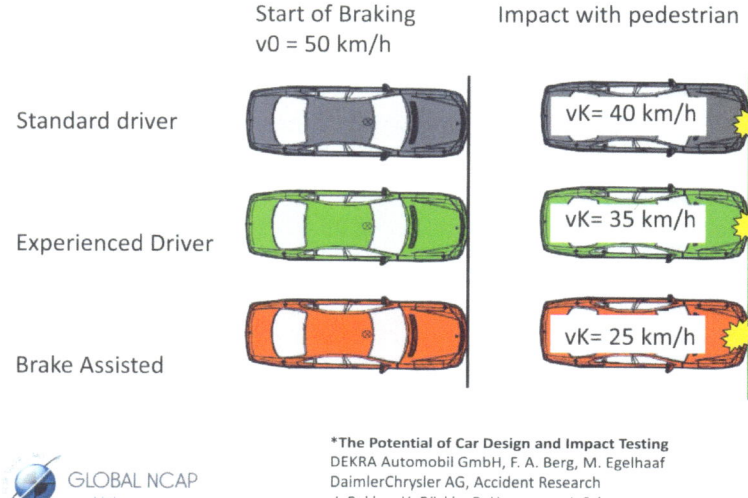

Figure 9.1(a) Potential collision speed reduction with AEB for drivers having different levels of experience (Source: Ward 2014)

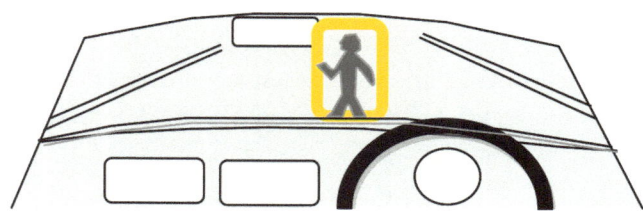

Figure 9.1(b) Concept – driver's view when approaching a pedestrian (Source: Based on Ward 2014)

AEB has developed from commercial research and applications of autonomous cruise control of vehicles since 1995, when a forward-looking collision avoidance system was offered on selected Mitsubishi vehicles. Others followed, including Toyota with radio detection and ranging (RADAR) cruise control in 1997 and a low speed 'tracking control' in 2000. The current form of AEB was initiated in 2003, and research and applications by various 'luxury' brands of cars have led to some installation and improvements.

Although some manufacturers have marketed their AEB systems under different names, the European New Car Assessment Programme (Euro NCAP) AEB Fitment Survey (2012) found that AEB technology was available on 21% of vehicles sold in Europe, even though potential accident savings would be up to 27% of the total. For most manufacturers AEB is still in the development stage and exact details of each system may vary and may not be available due to commercial reasons. Most systems use RADAR for inter-urban higher speeds in the 200 m range or LIDAR (Light Detection and Ranging Sensor) for AEB City in low-speed driving and a 6-8 m range.

Further studies (Rosen et al. 2013) indicate that for pedestrian accidents, with an activation rate of 65%, the average collision speed decreased from 32 km/h without AEB to 22 km/h with the system. This yielded an estimated reduction of fatally/severely injured pedestrians by 48%/42%. Thus, even moderate reductions of average collision speed were very effective. However, imposing a cut-off speed at 60 km/h had only a minor effect on average collision speed while the effectiveness dropped markedly. Variables such as lighting conditions, initial speed, field of view (FoV) of the sensing devices and other factors will affect the results.

Continuing development has resulted in improved sensors and related equipment, thereby aiding the detection and, importantly, identification of pedestrian movements as a vehicle approaches. These later developments are complicated; whereas vehicles following each other have relatively predictable trajectories and provide a substantial physical 'target' for detection, the movement of pedestrians is much more varied. For instance a pedestrian may stop suddenly before entering the carriageway, step out from behind a parked vehicle, walk slowly or run and present large variations in physical shape and size.

System Categories

Euro NCAP has grouped crash avoidance systems into three main categories: City, Inter-Urban, and Pedestrian, as shown in Figure 9.2. Systems may fall into just one category, or may meet the requirements of all three.

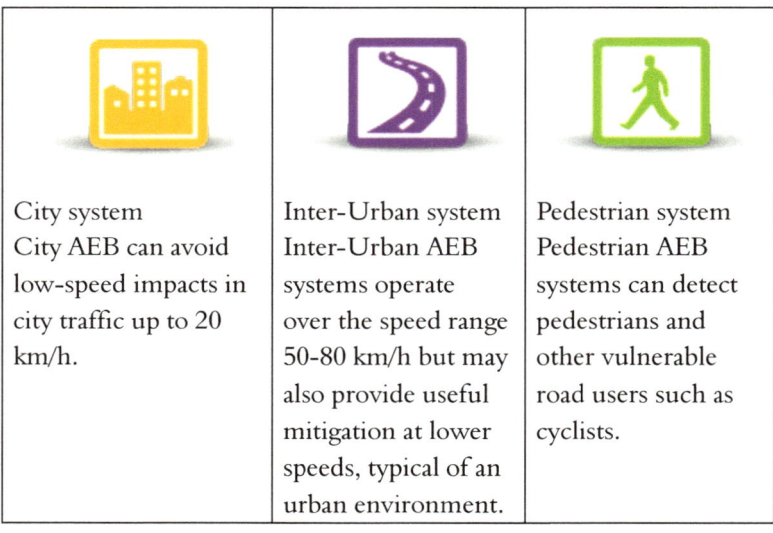

City system	Inter-Urban system	Pedestrian system
City AEB can avoid low-speed impacts in city traffic up to 20 km/h.	Inter-Urban AEB systems operate over the speed range 50-80 km/h but may also provide useful mitigation at lower speeds, typical of an urban environment.	Pedestrian AEB systems can detect pedestrians and other vulnerable road users such as cyclists.

Figure 9.2 AEB System categories (Source: Euro NCAP 2014)

City systems are those which can avoid an impact by autonomous braking at speeds up to 20 km/h where 80% of all whiplash injuries occur. These systems look for the reflectivity of a typical vehicle and so are not sensitive to pedestrians or roadside furniture.

Inter-urban systems do more than only warn the driver and also operate over the speed range 50-80 km/h. These systems are designed to see other road traffic including, in some cases, motorcycles and trucks. A potential advantage of RADAR sensors is their ability to function in all weathers and lighting conditions.

Pedestrian and other vulnerable road user (VRU) systems, as indicated earlier, are increasingly the focus of AEB development. Images from a forward-looking sensor system and camera in the vehicle are analysed to identify shapes and characteristics typical of humans. The forward-looking sensor system and camera are usually mounted at the rear-view mirror and are connected to an electronic control unit and the brake system. The camera combined with RADAR is known as sensor fusion. New technologies are entering the market which use infra-red and thus can operate in very low light.

Performance of AEB systems depends on a number of characteristics. For the sensor this includes a field of view (FoV), range of VRU detection, image-gathering rate and processing time. Vehicle characteristics include brake deceleration rate, time to maximum deceleration, maximum lateral distance from car path from VRU and cut-off speed of car above which AEB was not activated. The AEB would not be activated if the driver already braked harder than the AEB system itself. In effect, then, the AEB system is activated if, and only if, the following six requirements are satisfied:

- VRU visible and within sensor FoV and range
- Car is expected to collide with VRU
- VRU within a 'trigger' width which will activate the response
- Predicted time to collision is less than that under maximum AEB braking
- Driver decelerated slower than AEB
- Car speed is less than the maximum permitted for the with AEB system

Pedestrian avoidance or collision mitigation is achieved by sensing and calculating how pedestrians are moving relative to the path of the vehicle to determine whether they are in danger of being struck. If so, the AEB system applies full braking power to stop the car and, at the same time, it may issue a warning to the driver. Predicting human behaviour is difficult and the algorithms – the inputs, calculation and analysis sequence – used in pedestrian detection systems are complex. The system must be able to react properly to a valid threat but must not apply the brakes where there is no danger, e.g. where a pedestrian is walking to the edge of the footway but then stops to allow the car to pass. Examples of AEB application are shown in Figure 9.3.

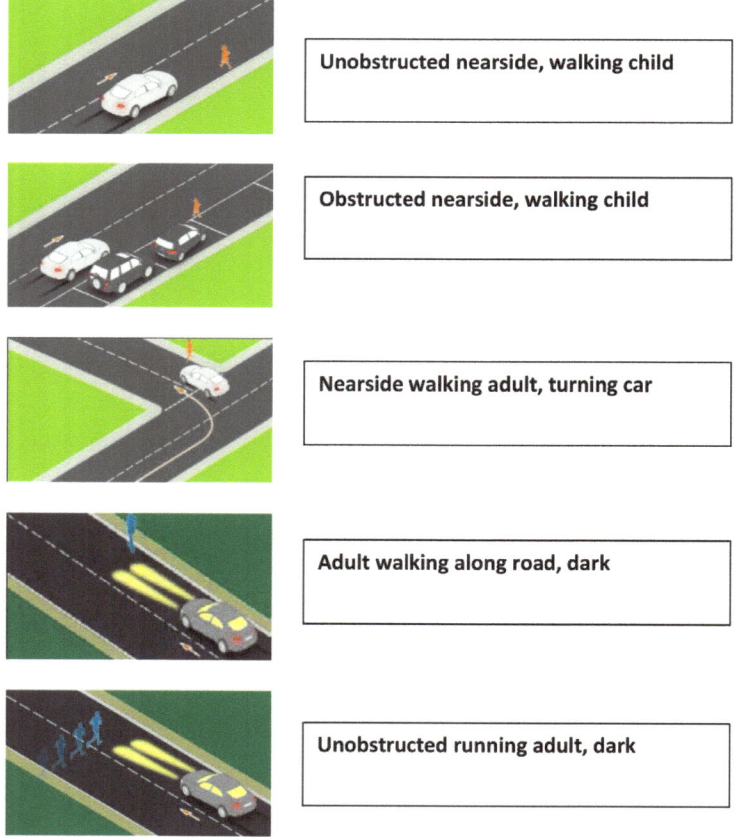

Figure 9.3 Examples of potential AEB collision avoidance and mitigation cases (Source: Euro NCAP 2014)

Pedestrians move in many ways when leaving the footway. A brief summary of the percentages of pedestrians' actions to determine an approximate breakdown of trajectories as a basis for examining potential scenarios for test speeds of between 10 km/h and 60 km/h is as follows (Avery 2013):

- Pedestrian walks into carriageway from nearside 51%
- Pedestrian walks from behind obstruction, e.g. a parked car 14%
- Pedestrians runs out from driver's right hand side 9%
- Pedestrian walks along carriageway in the dark 3%
- Pedestrian walks out into path of turning car 6%

Major features of the sensing and trigger widths (the latter being the maximum lateral distance from the car path to the pedestrian at which braking is activated) are shown in Figure 9.4.

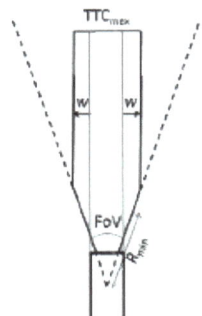
Fig. 2a. Specification of sensor system and parameters for decision algorithm. The area bounded by the solid contour was the trigger area.

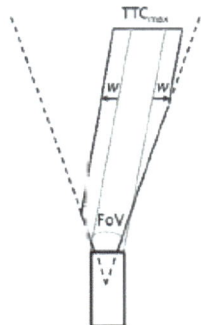
Fig. 2b. When the car turned, the predicted car path was in the momentary direction of travel of the vehicle front.

Figure 9.4 Features of sensor system for detecting pedestrians: (a) vehicle proceeding in a straight line and (b) vehicle turning a corner (Source: Rosen 2013)

TTC = Maximum time to collision
W = Trigger width – the maximum lateral distance from the car path to the pedestrian at which braking is activated
FoV = Field of view of the sensor

Although much work has been completed in developing AEB, several important concerns remain in its application (Rosen 2013). Essentially, because unwanted activation is undesirable due to being annoying or even posing a safety threat to the occupants, AEB is currently likely to be limited in its operating times and/or deceleration levels by user choice. Also, some systems may not operate successfully in darkness and at high speeds. With nearly 50% of pedestrian fatalities occurring at impact speeds of greater that 60 km/h (40 mph) and nearly 60% occurring at night, dusk or dawn, solutions to these limitations are being investigated but await satisfactory resolution.

Collision Reduction

As noted earlier, AEB has been predicted to offer a big reduction in the number and severity of pedestrian injuries. A combination of the AEB system with driver warning devices, and possibly also autonomous emergency steering, is scheduled for implementation and evaluation by consumers.

Estimated potential personal injury and damage savings based on the Association of British Insurers (ABI) motor claims statistics crashes to 2018, and models of AEB and electronic stability control (ESC) fitment rates for UK vehicles indicate that approximately 800,000 crashes could be prevented between 2012 and 2018, as indicated in Figure 5. Increasingly, motor vehicle insurers are reducing premiums for customers who install AEB systems, although the extent to which pedestrians are protected by the various systems varies.

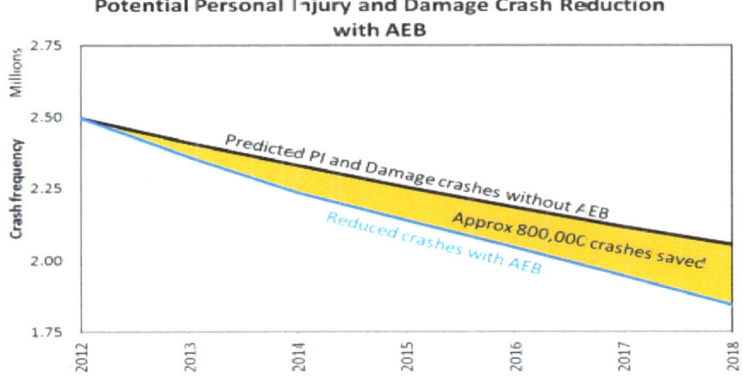

Figure 9.5 Potential injury and damage reduction with AEB (Source: Avery 2013)

Real-world performance data suggests that such crash avoidance systems can reduce accidents by up to 27% and can thus lead to a significant reduction in injuries.

Euro NCAP believes that AEB systems offer a considerable safety potential. Their assessment is included in the rating scheme from 2014 onwards, and tests have been developed to allow the performance of City and Inter-Urban systems to be compared. Euro NCAP has also repeated its AEB fitment survey, originally conducted in June 2012, to establish which systems are currently in the market and the extent to which they are made available by manufacturers. Euro NCAP summarises its conclusions as follows:

- Active safety – the ability to avoid a crash in the first place.
- Advance Driver Assistance Systems (ADAS) offer huge potential benefits.
- Autonomous Emergency Braking (AEB) appears to be the most important and significant.
- Real-world data shows current generation systems are reducing crashes by 27% (Volvo).

- Next generation of systems will offer bigger potential with most manufacturers introducing systems.
- Not all systems perform the same; some are more relevant for low-speed crashes and capable of directly addressing whiplash.
- There is a continuing need for performance tests to measure system efficacy.
- AEB tests under development using real-world crash scenarios, designed to measure system performance and relevance.
- Test procedures will be proposed to Euro NCAP for consideration as the basis of new test procedures to be introduced by 2013 – to address car-to-car and car-to-pedestrian injuries.
- UK insurance group rating intends to recognise AEB from 2013.

The benefits of AEB are being increasingly recognised. At a recent UK parliamentary meeting it was stated that (King 2014) the Government should give incentives for people to buy safer cars in the same way that incentives have been given for greener cars; according to King every now and then a new safety technology comes along that is worthy of widespread uptake as it will save lives. We have seen this with seatbelts, airbags, antilock brakes, electronic stability control and now we have the chance to embrace Autonomous Emergency Braking (AEB). Often such technologies are expensive at first and therefore only taken up by safety pioneers or those who can afford top end cars. We need to encourage car buyers, including fleet buyers, to specify AEB when choosing new cars.

King further stated:

> "We need to encourage manufacturers to make AEB available further down their model ranges and we need to encourage car buyers, including fleet buyers, to specify AEB when choosing new cars. As the Government has a good record of giving incentives to encourage the uptake of greener cars, we would like to see such incentives expanded to safer

cars. Our own motoring panel survey of 24,351 drivers clearly shows that the uptake of AEB would double if the Government was to provide a £500 cash incentive to those buying a car with AEB. More cars with AEB should mean fewer crashes, fewer injury claims and lower premiums."

Other relevant details concerning AEB include:

- 22% (22% male, 22% female) of car buyers are fairly or very likely to choose and pay for AEB as a £1,000 optional extra.
- This rises to 45% (43% male, 49% female) fairly or very likely to choose AEB as an option if the Government were to provide a £500 cash incentive to buy a car with AEB.
- The idea of the cash incentive seems to appeal particularly to younger drivers, with 60% of 18-24 year olds and 48% of 25-34 year olds fairly or very likely to choose AEB as an option if the Government were to provide a £500 cash incentive to buy a car with AEB.
- Although AEB is a general term for Autonomous Emergency Braking systems, different car manufacturers use their own names, for example Volvo's City Safety, Ford's Active City Stop and Volkswagen's City Emergency Braking are all AEB systems.
- AEB is already standard fit on some models but more widely available as an optional extra, often bundled with other Advanced Driver Assistance Systems. On average AEB is currently estimated to cost around £1,000 as an option on new cars.
- It is estimated that fitting a car with AEB would bring its insurance premiums down by 10%.
- AEB has the potential to save more than 1,200 lives and prevent 136,000 casualties over 10 years.
- UK insurance claims data shows an 18% reduction in the frequency of third party injury claims for cars fitted with AEB.
- 550,000 whiplash claims annually in the UK cost £2 billion, adding £90 to the average car insurance premium.
- 23% of new cars on sale today have AEB as optional or standard fit.
- Less than 10% of cars sold have AEB specified.

Clearly, the benefits of AEB in reducing vehicle/pedestrian collisions are considerable. A cautionary note is that automation essentially enables drivers to become "hands and feet free" but not "mind free" during vehicle operation (Banks et al. 2013). They mention that "automation may introduce additional complexity into the driving task by placing increasing pressure on drivers to monitor both the environment and behaviour of vehicle sub-systems". Much remains to be done in terms of technological advancement and human factors investigation in order to evaluate and develop the full potential of AEB and its promise of reducing pedestrian casualties.

Driverless Vehicles

A separate yet allied development from Euro NCAP is the 'driverless' vehicle. Developed recently with impetus from Google (Google 2016) and others, this currently experimental vehicle shows considerable promise in avoiding obstacles while completely automated. Clearly, the 'driverless' aspect completely removes the human and associated uncertainty from the driving task. However, the practicalities of its development are likely to continue for some time and hinge on the speed and location of operation and technicalities, including reliability of radio and electronic equipment.

Clearly, if vehicles can be developed to a stage where drivers are no longer required, much of the material in earlier chapters of this book will be less relevant. The assumption is that when vehicles are truly 'driverless' and assuming that pedestrians will still be present on most urban road systems, cars will need to have the ability to avoid pedestrians as, in the same way, ideally, a driver would do. So if a pedestrian, for example, had collapsed in the carriageway ahead of the car, the car would come to a stop.

Much of the existing challenge of developing a driverless vehicle appears to result from programming assuming that the vehicle behaves as it legally should, whereas many road users, including pedestrians, often (knowingly or unknowingly) commit 'minor' infractions. Other issues such as matters of a non-technical nature such as collision liability and insurance may prove to be even greater challenges.

A particular example is where a police officer signals a vehicle to proceed through a red signal, whereas the vehicle would stop because the signal would be identified as requiring a stop and the officer would be identified as a pedestrian unless the car's programming was able to distinguish the officer's uniform. This leads to the assumption that a driver should be present to override the automation, but this negates the intention of the programming and assumes that the driver is constantly alert – thereby defeating one of the original intentions of the 'driverless' concept, i.e. to avoid collision resulting from a driver's inattention.

Nevertheless, much has been accomplished during the research on the 'driverless' concept and it is possible that many of the ideas can contribute to the development of AEB-equipped vehicles, although the truly 'driverless' vehicle itself may be some decades in the future. British Government funding and interest are assisting development (Department for Transport 2015), and efforts are being made to assist both commercial and publicly sponsored projects.

Implementation

Recognition of the needs and advantages of AEB is made in a number of publications including *Which* magazine (2016) and *Working Together to Build a Safer Road System* (Department for Transport (DfT) 2015). Both refer to the present high cost to consumers under present 'bundling' with other options. The latter states: "Our challenge as a government is to promote consumer awareness of these life-saving innovations, encourage motorists to purchase the technologies and promote their adoption within car fleets and commercial organisations."

However, the level of enthusiasm of car buyers for purchase of AEB systems is informative; a random perusal of a week's newspaper motoring sections indicated that the preferred options in new cars included: gold stripe highlights to the sides of the car; child's TV for rear seats; racing alloy wheels; wood veneer panelling; heated seats; darkened windows; multi-speaker stereo; and personal logo dash emblems. AEB? – evidently some way to go. Perhaps mandatory installation and use of AEB systems in a similar way to that adopted for the life-saving seatbelts in motor vehicles could be the answer.

★

> *Although many aspects of development and application are being investigated, the likelihood of reducing vehicle/pedestrian accidents beyond the latest estimate of 27% is evidence of AEB's potential. As these matters continue to be explored and ways forward proposed, the potential for reducing pedestrian accidents is promising. Its installation in more vehicles should markedly reduce accidents as long as human factors such as over-reliance on the system do not reduce its effectiveness. Yet reduced cost and/or increased publicity will be necessary to induce the public to equip its vehicles with this life-saving technology. Failing this, mandatory installation may be necessary. "A golden age for pedestrians" (Mother Jones 2012) may be somewhat optimistic yet the possibilities, if realistic, are awe-inspiring and intriguing.*

References

Avery, Mathew (2013) *AEB Test Development*. Merida RCAR.

Banks, Victoria A., Neville A. Stanton and Catherine Harvey (2013) *Sub-Systems on the Road to Vehicle Automation: Hands Free But Not 'Mind' Free Driving*. Safety Science, Elsevier.

Department for Transport (DfT) (2015) *The Pathway to Driverless Cars, Summary Report*. PDF, UK.gov. Website accessed 2016.

Department for Transport (DfT) (2015) *Working Together to Build a Safer Road System. British Road Safety Statement*. London

Drum, Kevin (2012) *Driverless Cars Will be a Boon to Pedestrians. Mother Jones* magazine, San Francisco.

European New Car Assessment Programme (2014) http//euroncap.com/results/aeb.aspx. Accessed 6 February 2014.

European New Car Assessment Programme AEB Fitment Survey (2012) *Fifteen Years for Safer Cars: AEB Fitment Survey*. Presentation given at the 15th Anniversary Event, Brussels, 13 June 2012. Available at: http://prezi.com/wrid.

Google (2016) *Google Self Driving Car Project*. Website accessed March 2016.

King, E. (2014) Edmund King, Automobile Association (AA) president, speaking at a briefing in the House of Commons on Tuesday 25 March parliamentary meeting, organised by the Thatcham Research campaign 'Stop the Crash'. London.

Rosén, Erik, Jan-Erik Källhammer, Dick Eriksson, Matthias Nentwich, Rikard Fredriksson, Kip Smith (2010) *Pedestrian Injury Mitigation by Autonomous Braking*. Paper Number 09-0132. Autoliv Research, Sweden.

Rosén, E. (2013) *Autonomous Emergency Braking for Vulnerable Road Users*. IRCOBI Conference 2013 (IRC-13-71).

Ward, D. (2014) *Pedestrian Safety Developments in Crash Worthiness and Crash Avoidance*. 19th Meeting of the UN Road Safety Collaboration Convene Centre, 9 April 2014.

Which Ltd. Magazine (May 2016) *Autonomous Emergency Braking*.p.36. Hertford UK.

CHAPTER 10

VEHICLE DESIGN IMPROVEMENTS

Softening the impact

Extensive efforts have made vehicles safer for the occupants in the event of collision. Beginning with seat belts and their use – both now mandated on all vehicles – car design now features 'crumple zones' to absorb crash energy and protect driver and passengers. Progress on protecting pedestrians in vehicle/pedestrian collisions has been much slower. Belatedly, research and initial steps at designing and selling vehicles which absorb the energy of a pedestrian contact has led to big improvements. Other technologies associated with vehicle design which assist in avoiding a collision, including intelligent speed assistance, daytime running lights and rear blind zones, is also evident. Following a brief description of the mechanism of typical vehicle/pedestrian collisions, most of this chapter describes the European Commission's New Car Assessment Programmes (Euro NCAP) which rate and publicise the safety features of vehicles. This system is intended to assist consumers in selecting vehicles which help to reduce pedestrian casualty severity. Yet expenditure on vehicles which can save pedestrians' lives and injuries is disappointing, leading to the conclusion that more persuasive methods of equipping the vehicle fleet with pedestrian-saving features, and encouraging their purchase, may be appropriate.

★

What Happens in a Pedestrian/Vehicle Collision?

Most such crashes involve frontal impacts. Figure 10.1 summarises the contact points between the pedestrian and the car during a crash. Note that during car-pedestrian contact, the whole body wraps around the front of the car. An adult pedestrian is typically 'run under' rather than 'run over' by the striking car (WHO 2013).

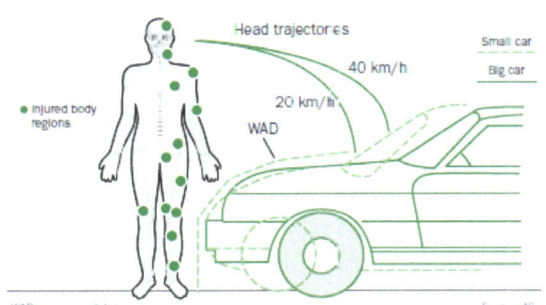

Note: The point at which a vehicle hits a pedestrian will vary depending on the height of a car as well as the height of the pedestrian. For example, a larger vehicle may hit the head of a child pedestrian because he or she is short.

Figure 10.1 Distribution of injuries on the body of a pedestrian in a frontal car-pedestrian collision (Source: WHO 2013)

To estimate the risk of injury in the event of a vehicle striking an adult or child, Euro NCAP carries out tests on the most important vehicle front-end parts such as the bonnet and windscreen, the bonnet leading edge and the bumper. The tests help to develop the energy-absorbing ability of the bumpers, deformation clearances to 'hard' features, and moving protection systems such as pop-up bonnets and external airbags.

Subsystem Tests

Assessing effective pedestrian protection using a full dummy is difficult. Although controlling the point of impact of the bumper against the pedestrian's leg is possible, it is impossible to control where the head will subsequently strike. To overcome this problem, individual component tests are used. A legform test assesses the protection afforded to the lower leg by the bumper, an upper legform test assesses the leading edge of the bonnet, and child and adult headform tests are used to assess the bonnet-top area.

Lower Legform   Upper Legform   Headform

Figure 10.2 Forms of pedestrian frontal collision (Source: WHO 2013)

Vehicle Design Features to Reduce Collision Severity

Basic frontal area design of the vehicle can decrease the severity of injuries. For example, protection can be improved with pedestrian friendly bumpers, which deform when they hit a pedestrian's leg. Protection is improved if the leg is impacted lower down, away from the knee, and if the forces are spread over a longer length of leg. For the leading edge of the bonnet, removal of unnecessarily stiff structures can reduce the extent of the injury. To protect the head, the top area of the bonnet must be able to deflect. Enough clearance must be provided above the engine parts beneath, which would stop this deflection. On some types of vehicles the packaging in the engine compartment can be altered to create this clearance, and other vehicles may use inflatable or energy-absorbing layers to achieve this space.

Deployable features which activate on impact can also reduce the effects of collision. Such features include a 'pop-up' bonnet designed to lift in a crash with a pedestrian to create more space to absorb the head impact and thus reduce the severity of the injury. Most systems on the market comprise contact sensors in the front bumper area of the car in combination with bonnet lifters such as springs, a pyrotechnic charge, or an external airbag. On vehicles equipped with such a protection system headform tests are carried out on the fully or partially deploying bonnet if the manufacturers can show that the sensors can trigger the system for the pedestrian stature, which is hardest to detect (often a young child), and that the system response time is fast enough to provide full protection before the head would contact the bonnet. The design must also provide adequate levels of protection just below trigger thresholds (the collision's contact force which activates the deployment) and at higher speeds, in order to provide a design which operates if conditions are slightly different from those predicted.

Safety Ratings

Safety ratings may be viewed as numerical tools for evaluating road traffic safety quality and potential for improvement (DaCoTA 2012, p. 4). The ratings in use either predict safety outcomes for given vehicle designs or provide a retrospective assessment based on crash data. Euro NCAP released a separate rating for pedestrians valid from 1997 to 2009. As of 2009, the pedestrian score has become an integral part of the overall rating scheme. For pedestrian protection Euro NCAP's results in this rating are achieved through state of the art legform, upper legform and child/adult headform tests which are more stringent than the legislative tests coming into force for all new EU-registered vehicles in 2015 (DaCoTA 2012, p. 5). The original pedestrian protection rating was based on adult and child headform tests and two legform tests. To get a good overall rating, vehicles must achieve a satisfactory pedestrian protection score. In order to encourage further progress Euro NCAP will require from 2012 a minimum 60% score in the pedestrian tests for new cars to receive a 5-star rating (DaCoTA 2012, p. 37).

As well as helping vehicle fleet buyers and individual consumers to buy cars which are safer for pedestrians, the impartial and objective information provided by safety rating systems is designed for use by policymakers, employers, road and vehicle planners, engineers and operators, road safety professionals, practitioners and economists. The ratings can help in establishing, implementing and monitoring of road safety targets, strategies and interventions. Also, global and European goals require greater attention than before to the provision of a safer network and vehicles, better emergency care systems and compliance by users with key safety rules, as well as meaningful shared responsibility and partnerships on the part of road system providers.

Euro NCAP: Safety Results

Pedestrian protection sub-system tests are carried out to replicate crashes involving child and adult pedestrians where impacts occur at 40 km/h (25 mph). Assessment of the various vehicle elements consider:

- the legform test – protection afforded to the lower leg by the bumper;
- the upper legform test – the leading edge of the bonnet and child and adult; and,
- headforms – the bonnet top area.

Impact sites are then rated fair, weak and poor.

A recent Swedish study (Strandroth et al. 2011) found significant correlation between Euro NCAP pedestrian score and injury outcome in real-life car-to-pedestrian crashes. The results showed a significant reduction of injury severity for cars with better pedestrian scoring, although cars with a high score could not be studied, due to lack of cases. The reduction of risk of serious medical impairment for average-performing cars vs. low-performing cars was, for example, 38% vs 10%. These results applied to urban areas with speed limits up to 50 km/h (approximately 30 mph), although no significant reduction was found in higher speed zones (DaCoTA 2012, p. 38).

Comparisons between pedestrian injury severity in real-life crashes and Euro NCAP test results indicate that "Provided every car on German roads would comply with a standard of 22 Euro NCAP point score in pedestrian protection, an injury reduction potential of 6% of fatalities and 9% seriously injured pedestrians in passenger car impacts could be estimated."

Ratings and Scores

A Safety Rating Advisory Committee (SARAC) survey of Euro NCAP ratings in Spain and Sweden concluded that Euro NCAP needed to be promoted more widely and effectively for it to play a higher role in fleet purchasing decisions and to encourage fleet managers to develop purchase policies which include specific safety criteria. The postal and telephone survey also concluded that both members of the public and fleet purchasers needed to be educated about sources of information about vehicle safety. Price and reliability seem to be more important than safety in the purchasing decisions of fleet management (DaCoTA 2012, p. 39).

Euro NCAP's ongoing strategy recognises the importance of informing the public about vehicle safety. It states its intention to support and better coordinate its activities with its member organisations and others interested in consumer safety. Also, it intends to carry out clear target-setting and periodic monitoring of how well its rating system is helping to reduce pedestrian and other deaths and injuries. So far the results in these respects are unclear.

Euro NCAP ratings comprise scores in each of the individual four areas (adult, child, pedestrian and safety assistance). The top achievers by category identified by Euro NCAP in the 2010 tests are shown in Table 10.1.

Table 10.1. Top achievers' scores in Euro NCAP tests 2010 (Source: Based on DaCoTA 2012)

Euro NCAP vehicle class	Star rating	Adult score	Child score	Pedestrian score	Safety assistance score
Executive category	5★	95%	83%	78%	100%
V small family category	5★	97%	85%	63%	86%
Supermini category	5★	93%	80%	71%	86%
Small off-road 4×4 category	5★	93%	86%	49%	86%
Small MPV category	5★	89%	75%	69%	86%

When a decision to purchase a particular car has to be made, the NCAP system can offer some guidance as to which cars offer protection in certain areas. For example, the pedestrian protection scores for large family cars varied from 54% to 80%. An example of Euro NCAP Crash Test Results for a selected typical five-door estate (Euro NCAP 2014) is shown in Figure 10.3, indicating a score of 66% for pedestrian protection. The excerpt for this pedestrian-related score states:

> The bumper scored maximum points for its protection of pedestrians' legs. However, the front edge of the bonnet scored no points, providing poor protection to the pelvis region. Tests on the bonnet surface revealed predominantly good or adequate levels of protection to the head of a struck pedestrian, with poor results recorded only on the stiff windscreen pillars. An Autonomous Emergency Braking

system is available as an option and can detect pedestrians as well as other vehicles, helping to avoid or to mitigate injuries to pedestrians and other vulnerable road users. As the system is not standard equipment, it was not included in the assessment.

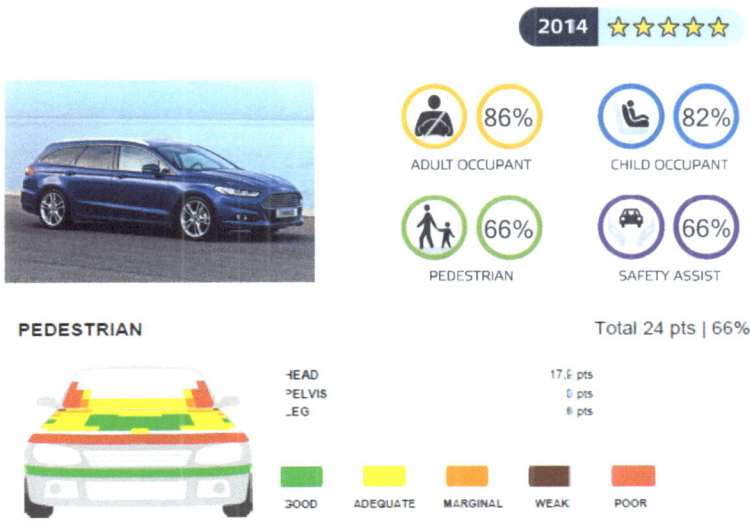

Figure 10.3 Excerpts from test results report, selected typical five-door estate (Source: Based on Euro NCAP 2014)

Examination of these reports indicates several areas which need further attention if they are to be of value to consumers and, resulting from their purchases, gradually ensuring that the vehicle fleet throughout Britain becomes more responsive to pedestrian safety; despite a particular car being awarded a 5-star rating its pedestrian score could be much lower than the score for other features.

Other Vehicle Safety Design Features

Vehicle design to encourage pedestrian safety in the event of a collision is a worldwide concern. However, vehicle design features which help to avoid a collision occurring in the first place are also, if not more, preferred. As well as the emphasis on activities in the UK and Europe, other countries are also experimenting with a variety of such design features. Briefly noted below are several summary indications of work being carried out by the Australian New Car Assessment Programme (ANCAP). Examples of the concerns particularly related to pedestrian safety include daylight running lights (Figure 10.4) and rear view blind spot mitigation (Figure 10.5).

Daylight running lights (DRLs) (Paine 2015). About 30% of struck pedestrians fail to see the car before the accident. Most of these happen during the daytime. Well-designed DRLs make the vehicle more conspicuous to pedestrians. Efficient LED systems will soon be available in Australia. With intelligent DRLs' light-sensitive switches the headlights automatically come on and DRLs switch off when the ambient light fades.

It is estimated that DRLs could prevent 12% of all pedestrian fatalities. Claims of vulnerable road users being 'masked' by vehicles with DRLs have been shown to be unfounded. Well-designed DRLs do not 'distract' other motorists – they instantly make the vehicle more conspicuous. This is an advantage because other road users can devote more time to detecting less conspicuous objects.

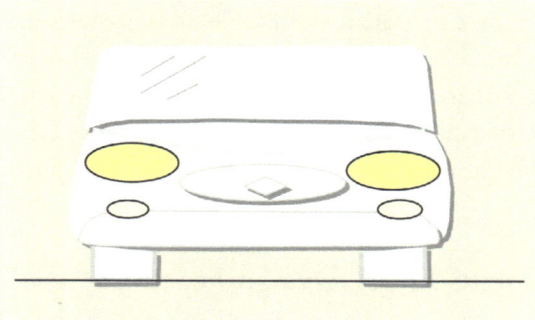

Figure 10.4 Daylight running lights and conspicuity (Source: Based on Paine, M., website accessed 2015)

Blind spot mitigation (Paine 2015). All vehicles have blind spots that pose a danger to pedestrians. The combination of a reversing motor vehicle and young children is a particular concern. In Australia typically 12 children die each year in low-speed vehicle accidents and many of these are reversing vehicles. The New South Wales Motor Accidents Authority (NSWMAA) has developed a range of countermeasures for this problem.

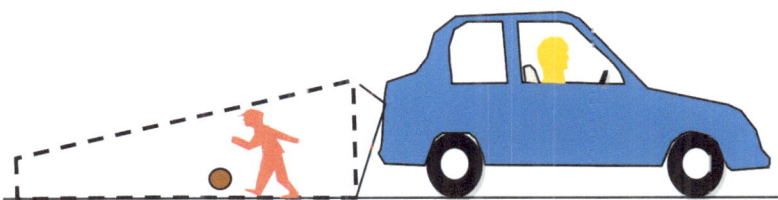

Figure 10.5 Blind spot mitigation (Source: Based on Paine, M., website accessed 2015)

The New South Wales Road Transport Authority (NSWRTA) has published a technical specification for assessing reversing aids such as cameras and ultrasonic sensors. It is stressed by all organisations that children need to be closely supervised by adults when near vehicles – technology can reduce but cannot eliminate the risk.

Prospects for Improved Pedestrian Protection

Improvements in the pedestrian safety performance of vehicles, while necessary and commendable, suffer from a problem: potential purchasers apparently are not clamouring for the pedestrian safety features to be installed and paid for. A high score on account of pedestrian safety features does not seem to influence a potential purchaser in buying that vehicle in preference to one which scores lower, other things, including price and operating cost, being equal.

A brief perusal of recent Sunday newspaper motoring and car sections highlighted key features which apparently, because of the attention given to them, might induce consumers to buy a particular car. No feature which could reduce the likelihood of a pedestrian's death or injury in a collision was mentioned.

★

> There is little doubt that the design of vehicles to reduce the physical trauma to pedestrians in a collision can greatly reduce the number of killed and injured pedestrians. Unfortunately, the lag in attention in vehicle design to pedestrian issues has resulted in a nationwide, sub-standard vehicle fleet in this respect. It is curious that, given the lethal nature of a moving vehicle compared to say that of a double barrel shotgun, the latter of which has a safety catch mechanism which lessens the probability of someone getting shot, there is no similar mechanism on the former which lessens the likelihood of a pedestrian getting killed or injured. *Strenuous efforts would seem appropriate to remedy this situation. Enhanced technical efforts encouraged by governmental and other signatories to Euro NCAP need to be made. The reporting of individual vehicle ratings and scoring to simplify and improve decision-making by consumers to improve pedestrian protection would seem to be desirable by government and manufacturers.* Seat belt installation was made mandatory to save the lives of vehicle occupants. Are pedestrians less important?

References

DaCoTA (2012) *Safety Ratings Deliverable 4.8r of the EC FP7 Project Da Cota*. Project co-financed by the European Commission Directorate General for Mobility & Transport 29/01/2013 www.dacota-project.eu.

European New Car Assessment Programme (2014) *The Best in Class Cars 2014*. European Commission, Brussels.

European New Car Assessment Programme. *Research, Design and Rating of Reduced Pedestrian Collision Systems*. Website accessed 29 March 2015.

Paine, M. *Pedestrian Protection Through Vehicle Design – Australian New Car Assessment Programme (ANCAP)*. Website accessed 2015.

World Health Organization (2013) *Pedestrian Safety: A Manual for Decision-makers and Practitioners*. Geneva.

CHAPTER 11

ACTIONS FOR IMPROVEMENTS

"Think global, act local" (Geddes 1915)

Government agencies associated with road safety, including pedestrian travel, have responsibilities for local concerns and for the longer-term changes in official design guidance usually issued for national application. Quasi-governmental and private groups also issue analyses and often actively campaign for improvements. After briefly considering central government the review, which mainly addresses local government, is based upon RoSPA's publication *A Guide for Local Councillors in England.* This recognises that much of the effectiveness of road safety programmes and actions stems from the involvement of local councillors and safety officers. Also, the pedestrians' interest group, Living Streets, has produced a 'toolkit' with much practical advice for achieving local pedestrian safety, and this too is featured here. Finally, a brief description is made of a local pedestrians' interest group.

★

Central Government

Central government sets the regulatory framework, provides resources for local government, data collection and publishing, vehicle standards, motorway and trunk road management, commissioning research and education, setting licensing requirements and laws, penalties and guidance such as the *Design Manual for Roads and Bridges (DMRB), Manual for Streets (MfS)* (2007) and the Highway Code.

The Department for Transport (DfT) published its *Strategic Framework for Road Safety* (2011) setting out its approach to reducing death and injury on Britain's roads, and the range of measures by which it, and others, will do so. It includes a Road Safety Action Plan and a wide range of performance indictors against which progress will be measured. The *Strategic Framework for Road Safety* also reflects the Government's overall policy of 'localism', which aims to allow local authorities and local citizens to decide their own priorities for road safety in their areas, and to link their road safety agendas with other local agendas, such as public health and sustainable travel. Central government supports this by providing access to guidance and information to the public and to road safety professionals. For example, English highway authorities are required to publish casualty, collision and speed data for permanent fixed camera sites on their roads, and a website to allow local people to compare road safety performance in their area against other similar ones.

Local Government

Local government is the main delivery agent of road safety; local authorities have a statutory duty under Section 39 of the 1988 Road Traffic Act (DfT 1988) to "take steps both to reduce and prevent accidents". This involves the Secretary of State promoting road safety by: disseminating information or advice relating to the use of roads; requiring each local authority to prepare and carry out a programme of measures to promote road safety; carrying out studies of accidents and implementing measures to reduce them such as training, construction and maintenance of roads.

Upper tier local authorities (such as county councils, metropolitan district councils and unitary authorities) have legal responsibilities for highways and transportation in their area. Lower tier authorities (such as district councils) do not, but do help to deliver road safety services. London is a separate case; Transport for London (TfL) manages the Transport for London Road Network (TLRN),

London's traffic lights and transport services across the capital. The rest of London's road network is managed by London borough councils and the Common Council of London, each of which is a unitary authority. Trunk roads and motorways in England are managed by Highways England.

Every local highways authority has a road safety team or, in the case of some smaller unitary authorities, a road safety officer. Their role is to provide professional expertise to identify the causes of problems and to help to identify, develop and provide solutions for those problems.

Local highways authorities also have road safety engineering teams who seek to identify and implement road design and engineering solutions to road traffic casualties in their areas. The road safety education and engineering teams should work together, as well as in co-operation with other agencies, such as the police, fire and rescue service and others. Local authority officers also share knowledge and experience with each other across the country, in many ways, including through Road Safety GB, the Chartered Institution of Highways and Transportation (CIHT) and the Road Safety Knowledge Centre (www.roadsafetyknowledgecentre.org.uk).

Local authorities also have a duty to manage and maintain their road networks under Section 16 of the Traffic Management Act 2004. This act emphasises the 'expeditious' movement of traffic, the efficient use of the network and the avoidance, elimination or reduction of road congestion or other disruption to the movement of traffic on their road network or a road network for which another authority is the traffic authority. *Note that pedestrian traffic is not specifically mentioned separately, although pedestrians are classed as "traffic" in the 1988 Road Traffic Act.*

Town and parish councils may also acquire a more important role in road safety as emphasis on the local area develops, for example by funding speed indication devices, traffic calming or community schemes. Many highway authorities have already established forums to allow parish councils to request lower speed limits or improvements to road design. These represent important channels through which the wishes of local communities can be heard.

Local authorities that are a highway authority are responsible for highway maintenance, transport strategy and policy, including road safety, accident investigation and prevention, public transport and sustainable transport for their areas.

A Local Transport Plan (LTP) setting out strategy, targets and an implementation plan for improving transport in their community is required by local authorities in England (outside London). The Plan is used to apply for government funding for local transport needs, and should show how they intend to reduce the number of people being killed and injured on their roads. The LTP should include all road safety engineering, education, enforcement and encouragement activities planned for the next five years, including with other agencies. It should also review the effectiveness of the measures employed in any previous plan. Road safety managers are best placed to lead the development of the road safety part of the LTP. In London, each local authority produces a Local Implementation Plan (LIP) setting out how it will meet the Mayor of London's Transport Strategy.

Reliable data acquisition is essential before any road safety programme (engineering, education, enforcement or a combination) can be planned. Both local data usually collected by the police and national data and summaries (see Chapter 4) are of value, and are available to identify priority problem areas, roads and/or groups (e.g. young drivers) and to plan road safety programmes.

Published research can guide local road safety officers in setting their priorities and activities. Two useful organisations that provide access to a wide range of road safety research and good practice are the Road Safety Observatory and the Road Safety Knowledge Centre.

Road safety programmes designed from the analysis of this data and research may cover road safety education, engineering, enforcement or a combination of some or all of these approaches.

Some local authorities produce or commission reviews of their overall casualty situation or about particular groups of road users. For example, Cornwall Council and Plymouth University (2012) have produced a range of road safety reports to inform and support the Council's road safety education, engineering and enforcement initiatives.

Education, training and publicity at local level are designed to provide information, raise awareness and give advice on appropriate behaviour; they can also reinforce positive attitudes. All three activities aim to influence the behaviour of road users, by improving their knowledge of the causes and consequences of road crashes, improving their skills as road users and fostering positive attitudes towards behaving in a way that reduces the risk of causing or being involved in a road accident. Although road user education is incorporated within the Scottish schools' curriculum, it is currently an optional element in England and Wales, and so is dependent on local enthusiasm and commitment down to the level of each individual school and teacher.

The police enforce road traffic laws, but some areas, such as parking enforcement, are the responsibility of local authorities. The police also co-operate with other agencies, such as the Health and Safety Executive (2003) to investigate serious work-related road accidents. Roads policing supports and complements road safety education and engineering, and is an essential part of road safety. It: deters illegal, dangerous and careless behaviour on the road; identifies offenders; investigates the causes of crashes; and helps to educate and change the attitudes of road users.

Road Safety Partnerships operate across the country based around police force areas. Many started as Safety Camera Partnerships, and many are called Casualty Reduction Partnerships. They normally comprise local authorities, police, courts, fire and rescue service, the health authority and other bodies. Their main aim is to work together in a co-ordinated approach to reduce the number of casualties on the roads in the Partnership's area, and make the best use of their combined efforts and resources. Public health is an increasingly important partner for local authorities, especially through the local health and wellbeing boards.

Police and Crime Panels scrutinise the work of each Police and Crime Commissioner and make sure information is publically available. The Panels include a councillor from every local authority in the police force area. For more information, see *Police and Crime Panels: Guidance on Role and Composition*, published by the Local Government Association (LGA) and the Centre for Public Scrutiny (CfPS) (website accessed 10 February 2016). In London, Transport for London and the London local authorities have the power, under the Traffic Management Act 2003 (2004) and the London Local Authorities and Transport for London Act 2003, to take responsibility for the civil enforcement of a range of non-endorsable moving traffic offences.

Employers have duties under 'health and safety' law to assess and manage the risks faced and created by their staff when they are using the road for work. Some road traffic laws also have 'cause or permit' offences which can apply to employers. A high proportion of journeys made on the road are work-related (for example, delivering goods, driving to appointments), and it is estimated that between a quarter and a third of all road crashes involve someone using the road for work. Local authorities are also major employers themselves, and have many staff who drive, ride or walk on the road in order to do their jobs. Therefore, local authorities should have policies and measures to manage their own work-related road safety risks. *Driving at Work: Managing Work-Related Road Safety* (2003) is a free guide published by the Department for Transport and the Health and Safety Executive. Advice and free resources to help employers manage their occupational road risk are available from RoSPA.

Council members and staff face and create risks for themselves and everyone else using the road. Proactively managing these risks means that they are less likely to be exacerbated by work pressures, such as journey schedules that encourage speeding. Familiarity with the council's 'At-work Road Safety' or 'Managing Occupational Road Risk' policies, which should apply to all council staff, including contractors and elected members, will assist considerably in keeping people safe.

Other agencies and groups, both private and public, help to deliver road safety services, for example, national and local charities and associations such as RoSPA and other organisations. Driver and motorcyclist trainers play a significant role in helping people become safer drivers and riders and in providing refresher and advanced training. Youth organisations, e.g. Scouts, Brownies and others, often provide road safety courses and achievement awards. Many other groups help to improve road safety such as Cornwall Council and Plymouth University (2012) who address the needs and issues associated with young drivers.

Road safety engineers and urban designers use a wide range of measures to improve the safety of the road environment for all road users often as outlined in *Manual for Streets* (DfT 2007) and *Manual for Streets 2* (CIHT 2010). These measures can range from better road signs, markings and road surfaces to avoidance of street clutter, junction redesign, traffic calming schemes, 20 mph limits and zones, and improved walking or cycling facilities. Major road improvement schemes or Shared Space schemes may also be included. The objective of the road environment is to:

> **WARN** road users of any unexpected features or those requiring special attention
> **INFORM** road users about what is expected

GUIDE road users, making appropriate behaviour an easy choice

CONTROL road users as far as possible where conflicts may exist

FORGIVE error or inappropriate behaviour.

Other organisations, notably the Chartered Institution of Highways and Transportation (CIHT), provide useful guidance on planning and design of pedestrian facilities such as those by Mitchell and Bendixson (2015) and Philpotts (2015).

Safety engineers usually have an even greater impact on casualty reduction by undertaking area-wide or route-based safety schemes rather than focusing only on selected individual sites.

Road safety engineers also conduct road safety audits of existing roads and planned developments to identify problems and solutions. Their work is part of the overall safety effort in which other concerns such as maintenance and enforcement play critical roles, and in which policy on sustainable travel, and school crossings and school travel plans, are essential components.

Planning and development control is a longer-term measure available where a local authority is the local planning authority, and is responsible for regulating and controlling new developments within its boundaries. Officers and councillors decide whether or not proposals for new developments are acceptable.

The council must process and determine applications for planning permission, and regulate the schemes and developments which may be granted planning permission. This presents opportunities to anticipate and avoid potential road hazards, and to make walking and cycling, as well as driving, safer at the design stage – always the most effective (and cost-effective) way. It prevents problems before they arise, ensures that new road safety risks are not created and can also provide extra road safety measures to reduce the deleterious effects of increased traffic and changes in routes resulting from residential or commercial developments.

People or groups who participate in improving road safety can work with local councillors who have considerable opportunities for assisting in the process. An elected councillor can help to ensure that the local authority has a comprehensive local road safety strategy that is effective. In particular, the councillor can inform and influence the decisions through the cabinet or committee structure to ensure: that road safety resources are used to the best effect; that opportunities to improve safety on the road are not missed; and that any possible adverse effects are fully understood – including questioning acquired data to ensure that it is accurate and robust, and also to help present it to the public.

The councillor may also sit on other bodies which may have concerns about pedestrian facilities such as a school governing body or a health and wellbeing board, either as a representative of the authority or of the local community.

The interaction between human factors and road features has important implications for safety engineering and road user education, and highlights the need for engineers, road safety officers, roads police and others to work closely together. Understanding the human factors is part of the road safety officer's expertise and training. His or her role should be to provide that knowledge to the other disciplines by a combined problem-solving approach to highway design and accompanying campaigns and information. This enables the road user to be at the heart of design, education and enforcement. Councillors are in a unique position to enhance this co-operation and to become actively involved in making their roads safe.

Councillors can become aware of a problem because of complaints from constituents before they are reflected in the casualty statistics, and can bring this information to the notice of officers for further investigation. A challenge for councillors is how to respond to constituents' calls for action to prevent what they believe is an "accident waiting to happen" at a particular location. With limited resources, it is even more important to target road safety at real rather than perceived road safety problems. A perceived problem, however, may be a real barrier to people choosing to walk and cycle and, therefore, may justify action as part of the council's overall sustainable travel strategy.

The councillor's membership of the local scrutiny committee can enable the challenging of evidence and assumptions made by officers, as well as bringing partners together and looking at new and innovative ideas for reducing road accidents and casualties. Many other scrutiny committees across the country have looked at various aspects of road safety, for example the Centre for Public Scrutiny website (www.cfps.org.uk) can provide useful information.

Individual Actions for Change – a Toolkit

Complementing the advice to local councillors are actions which can be taken on traffic and safety issues by citizens of the area. The national organisation Living Streets takes an extensive interest in all pedestrian concerns and has published advice, including through a toolkit, on assisting local and national representatives on attaining improvements in pedestrian safety.

The toolkit addresses the process of planning, implementing and evaluating. It includes films with advice from Living Streets campaigners to assist. The remainder of this section is based on Living Streets' 'Make a Change – How to Take Action' (www.livingstreets.org.uk).

The first step is to identify the problem. To start, clarify the problem or issue. Example campaign issues may include: lack of a particular service in the community; traffic going too fast in the neighbourhood; or pavement parking.

Credibility is essential. Some questions include: What is the issue? What is the cause of the problem? Who is affected and how? Who has the power to make change happen? What change would you like to see? Has something similar happened elsewhere? Who can help you? Answering these questions will be essential before moving to the next stage. If possible collect evidence of the problem. You might consider:

- conducting a traffic survey to count the number of vehicles or the average speed of cars on your road;
- counting the number of steps to your nearest shop or the number of services available on your high street; and,
- undertaking a questionnaire to show how many other people agree with you.

There are many online resources to help in making a case. Living Streets has a range of resources that may be useful.

The second step is to start small and set the aims. Start talking and thinking about solutions to the problem. Positive messaging with the solution identified will show that your campaign is thoroughly thought-out and focused.

Many local campaigns will rely on targeting particular decision makers, individuals or groups. Think about who or what will influence them. These questions will help get you thinking about messaging: What is the call to action? Is the issue attention grabbing and urgent? Does the campaign message reflect this? What motivates your target? How will the change help or affect them? Have you worded the message positively with solutions identified? Is your message backed up by evidence?

Which groups to target and the means of communicating with them will be an ongoing concern. Decision makers will often be local councillors or council officials. A positive relationship, while being clear about the problem, is important and offering solutions will assist this relationship, even if the preferred solution may be different. Also, identify who influences your decision maker. It could be their constituents, the media, businesses, other councillors or other campaign groups. You can then approach these groups or individuals to strengthen your campaign.

Before collaborating with another group, consider whether you share a common vision, what resources they can provide and whether they have any similar experience. Do they have time to commit to your campaign? Relationships with the local media will be extremely useful when it comes to publicising the campaign. Local newspapers, radio stations and even television programmes will help. Local media may ask for updates and give a great deal of coverage, especially if there are similar issues in your area.

Local support can be obtained from the community by holding events and meetings, and also through social media. Specifically:

- Hold an event
- Run a stall at a local event
- Organise a meeting

You may wish to consider also having some 'take home' information for interested individuals. This should contain the campaign message, information on how to get involved and details of planned campaigning activities. Any materials should follow Living Streets guidelines. Consider also writing a blog, starting a Facebook group or posting updates on Twitter.

In engaging with black and minority ethnic (BME) and other diverse groups, the local authorities can help. Many now have a community involvement unit. One useful department within the local authority is the leisure department. Get involved by:

- asking for its list of groups and informal networks that represent ethnic minorities, refugee/asylum seekers and other excluded groups;

- visiting, listening and learning. People may not be receptive at first. However, it is important to be patient and persistent. Focus more on what you can offer them, not on what you want from them;
- attending meetings/events on an agreed date;
- at the meeting passing around a contact list form/template for people to put their details down; and,
- following up enquiries that people may have raised.

It is at this stage that the relationship process really begins. Think about ways that you can support the identified groups' work in their local community. It is critical not to lose the momentum and continue to build trust. In building trust, always be clear about what you have to offer the community; the contribution from minority communities, large segments of whom may depend on walking for daily activities, can be considerable.

Finally, as the campaign reaches a critical stage, an evaluation checklist can help to chart the continuing efforts. A possible checklist is as follows:

- What do you plan to achieve from the activity (survey, meeting, etc.) you are carrying out?
- Have you set measurable targets (e.g. numbers of people attending) and mechanisms for recording these?
- Would you be able to assess whether there is equal representation, e.g. whether you have only reached certain groups? What will you do to follow this up?
- Is it appropriate to have a mechanism for getting people's comments such as feedback forms, storyboards, etc? Have you put this in place?
- Are you planning any follow-up to tell people what the outcomes of their comments/views were?
- Does someone have clear responsibility for taking forward the views expressed to ensure that the activity has a successful outcome?
- What can be learnt in preparation for the next activity/event?

Further information on the means and resources useful in conducting a road safety campaign emphasising pedestrians' interests can be found on the Living Streets website.

[Author's note: Contact with the local road safety officer and police departments can be useful and informative, and can lend credibility to a campaign by providing factual data and experience of similar cases in other areas.]

Example of a Local Pedestrian Interest Group – Wirral Pedestrians Association

Local interest groups that are improving pedestrian facilities exist throughout the UK. An example of a local interest group formed in response to high pedestrian accident rates and the need for efforts to work closely with the local council and police is the Wirral Pedestrians Association. The Association has co-operated with police and other organisations to address many of the problems encountered by pedestrians in the Wirral area – problems which are also present throughout the UK.

★

> The ways of reducing accidents and improving pedestrian safety and mobility often depend on local action. *This review of local government's role in road safety, the approach that can be adopted by councillors and other local government staff and groups of individuals gives some idea of the scope of potential ways of achieving casualty reduction. The toolkit of Living Streets offers practical advice for action. The example of the Wirral Pedestrians Association (2012) provides a potential template for establishing a more formal and effective group which, by its actions, has obtained significant improvements in a number of cases within its area.*

References

Chartered Institution of Highways and Transportation (CIHT) (2010) *Manual for Streets 2 – Wider Application of the Principles.* Accessed at www.ciht.org.uk/en/publications.

Cornwall Council and Plymouth University (2012) *Implications for Education, Engineering and Enforcement Initiatives.* Accessed at www.cornwall.gov.uk/default.aspx?page=30370.

Cornwall Council and Plymouth University (2012) *Young Drivers: A Literature Review and Exploratory Analysis of Fatalities and Serious Injury Collisions in Relation to Young Drivers.* Plymouth, UK.

Department for Transport (1988) *The Road Traffic Act 1988.* Accessed at www.legislation.gov.uk/ukpga/1988/52/contents.

Department for Transport (2004) *Traffic Management Act 2004.* Accessed at www.legislation.gov.uk, 2015.

Department for Transport (2007) *Manual for Streets.* Thomas Telford. London.

Department for Transport (2011) *Strategic Framework for Road Safety.* London.

Department for Transport (2003) *London Local Authorities and Transport for London Act 2003.* Accessed at www.legislation.gov.uk/ukla/2003/3/contents.

Department for Transport & Health and Safety Executive (2003) *Driving at Work: Managing Work-Related Road Safety.* Accessed at www.hse.gov.uk/pubns/indg382.pdf.

Department for Transport (2012) *Reported Road Casualties in Great Britain 2011.* London.

Geddes, Patrick (1915) *Think global, act local. Cities in Evolution.* London: Williams.

Living Streets (Undated) *Make a Change – How to Take Action.* Accessed at www.livingstreets.org.uk.

Local Government Association and the Centre for Public Scrutiny (2011) *Police and Crime Panels: Guidance on Role and Composition.* Website accessed 10 February 2016.

Mitchell, K. and Bendixson, T. (2015) *Planning for Walking. Chartered Institution of Highways and Transportation (CIHT).* London.

Philpotts, M. (2015) *Designing for Walking. Chartered Institution of Highways and Transportation (CIHT).* London.

Royal Society for the Prevention of Accidents (2013) *A Guide for Local Councillors in England.* London.

The Centre for Public Scrutiny (Undated). Accessed at www.cfps.org.uk, March 2016.

UK Government (2004) *Traffic Management Act 2004.* Accessed at www.legislation.gov.uk/ukpga/2004/18/contents.

UK Government (2003) *London Local Authorities and Transport for London Act 2003.* Accessed at www.legislation.gov.uk/ukla/2003/3/contents/enacted.

Wirral Pedestrians Association (2012) *Constitution.* Website accessed March 2016. http://www.wirralpedestrians.org.uk.

Other Useful Publications

Department for Transport (2011) A Valuation of Road Accidents and Casualties in Great Britain in 2010. In *Reported Road Casualties in Great Britain: 2010 Annual Report*, https://www.gov.uk/government/uploads/system/uploads/attachment_data/file/9275/rrcgb2011-02.pdf.

Department for Transport (2012) Contributory Factors to Reported Road Accidents. In *Reported Road Casualties in Great Britain*. London.

Department of Health (2012) *A Short Guide to Health and Wellbeing Boards*. Accessed at www.healthandcare.dh.gov.uk/hwb-guide//index.cfm/manual-for-streets-2-wider-application-of-the-principles-2010.

Department of Health (2011) *Improving Outcomes and Supporting Transparency, Part 1: A Public Health Outcomes Framework for England, 2013-2016*. London.

Fire and Rescue Services Act 2004. Accessed at www.legislation.gov.uk/ukpga/2004/21/section/8.

Local Government Association and the Centre for Public Scrutiny. *Police and Crime Panels: Guidance on Role and Composition*. London.

Traffic Management Act 2004. Accessed at www.legislation.gov.uk/ukpga/2004/18/contents.

World Health Organization (2004) *World Report on Road Traffic Injury Prevention*. Geneva.

www.legislation.gov.uk/ukpga/2006/40/section.

Yass, I. (2010) *Delays Due to Serious Road Accidents*. RAC Foundation. Accessed at www.racfoundation.org/assets/rac_foundation/content/downloadables/road.

CHAPTER 12

PEDESTRIAN CASUALTY REDUCTION ESTIMATES

Improving safety – some numbers

A potentially useful intent of this book is to see how and to what extent pedestrian casualties can be minimised. Major causes of collisions with pedestrians such as speeding, alcohol use, inexperience and lack of attention by drivers were outlined in earlier chapters. Continuing awareness of these causes is, hopefully, anticipated to at least stabilise the numbers of deaths and injuries of people walking. Current and potential means of reducing accidents, through the use of 'black boxes' (or event data recorders (EDRs)), Autonomous Emergency Braking (AEB) and improved vehicle design were reviewed and numerical evidence of reductions due to these measures were highlighted. These three rapidly developing technological advances are the major sources of additional pedestrian casualty reductions estimated in this chapter.

It must also be remembered that current statistics on pedestrian casualties refer to people who were walking. As indicated earlier, especially in Chapter 4, the design of many pedestrian facilities is such that many people do not walk because they feel they cannot be in control of their own safety. They too are 'casualties' of the pedestrian system, in that they may suffer from lack of mobility and related health, wellbeing and economic problems. Research on the extent of this problem is sparse. But if approximately 12% of the population of 65 million people experience some form of disability then nearly 8 million people, plus children who are physically capable, are in fact continuing 'casualties' of our pedestrian system.

★

Estimation Methods

Any effort to predict future events as varied as the many ways of not killing and maiming pedestrians will necessarily be approximate. Given the unpredictability of governmental attention culminating in legislation mandating, for example, the standard installation in new vehicles of AEB (the equivalent of seat belts for vehicle occupants), this is perhaps not surprising.

Nevertheless, some indication of the effectiveness of various measures can provide the basis for achievable improvement programmes. The estimated reduction in casualties can thereby provide a more realistic basis for commitment to research and development by governmental and commercial interests, practical trials and, ultimately, a target for improvements. Such a target will, of course, be the subject of much speculation and the results subject to new developments as technological and legislative actions evolve.

Given the scarcity of factual information on the numerical reductions in casualties, estimates of future values are to a large degree speculative. One approach to obtaining an estimated figure when only minimal input data are available is to establish one or more 'scenarios' where input values are based on a 'what if' basis. In this approach, following review of the source, likelihood and level of certain inputs, a value is established, possibly judgmentally and/or following a consensus of people knowledgeable about the subject. This is the approach taken here, i.e. establishing apparently reasonable and conservative 'what if' input values which are then incorporated into a relatively simple arithmetic structure to obtain future estimates of future pedestrian casualties (Schoon 2015).

The numerical input values for calculating total reductions in this chapter are from two sources:

1. The current estimates developed by Mitchell and Allsop (2013) and described in Chapter 1, based on general ongoing

improvements to the year 2030, i.e. those related to the road safety improvement trends such as 20 mph speed limits, reductions in alcohol and substance abuse, attention to assisting young and inexperienced drivers and related measures.

2. Additional pedestrian casualty reduction estimates due to gradual implementation of three measures as the vehicle fleet is renewed to the year 2030. Implementation of such improvements is anticipated to have results on pedestrian casualties similar in the impacts of seat belt and vehicle design improvements mandated for vehicle occupants. The three measures are:

- *EDR*
- *AEB and*
- *Vehicle design improvements*

The calculation approach is to use the percentage improvements resulting from each of the three measures to numerically reduce the estimated number of accidents developed by Mitchell and Allsop for the year 2030 (termed the 'basic values' in the calculations below). These percentages are based on the values described in the relevant earlier chapters (8, 9 and 10).

The rationale for selecting the reduction percentages for each of the three measures is summarised below:

Event data recording (EDR). Speeding, drunkenness, carelessness and inattention are all behaviours of which a driver is aware and all entail risk of collision. If drivers are monitored by an EDR and can therefore be held accountable for their behaviour, they are less likely to engage in such a risk and consequently drive more carefully at all times that the EDR is operating. This is likely to result in reduced pedestrian casualties due to:

- collisions where only the driver is at fault, i.e. collisions with pedestrians who are behaving responsibly and correctly in accordance with rules, regulations and good conduct, such as correctly using a zebra crossing;

- collisions where both driver and pedestrian may be at fault, for example the driver going too fast when young children are playing unsupervised on the footway of a busy road.

In addition, if the EDR system is equipped with an e-call (emergency) function which is responsive to an injured pedestrian's need for urgent medical attention, the likelihood of death or the level of injury will be reduced.

Current reductions in collisions resulting from installation and use of EDR described and referenced in Chapter 8 are:

- 62% accident reduction (DriveCam 2004)
- 28.1% reduction in collisions (SAMOVAR 2007)
- 20% reduction in collisions (all Berlin police radio patrol vehicles are now fitted with EDRs) (SARAC 2004 c)
- 20% reduction in crashes in car, truck and coach fleets (SARAC 2004 c)
- 38% reduction in accidents and in unsafe driving practices and 82% savings in personal and vehicle fleet costs (RoSPA 2013).

Where a pedestrian in a collision is at fault either through inattention or incapacity, or if a vehicle is being driven more carefully, the collision is likely to be less severe.

> In view of the foregoing, and reflecting the fact that with the introduction of AEB the driver may rely more on its presence, the effectiveness of the EDR may be somewhat diminished; *the 'what if' percentage reduction assumed for the EDR implementation scenario is 20%, thereby reducing the basic value to 80% of its projected amount.*

Autonomous Emergency Braking (AEB)

AEB, irrespective of the driver's actions, will reduce the effects of the driver's speeding, drunkenness, carelessness and inattention mentioned above. Unlike EDR, because the AEB can act on behalf of the driver, there can be a tendency for the driver to: (a) drive more aggressively knowing that emergency situations will be accommodated by the AEB application of brakes and/or steering and: (b) pay less attention to the driving task, again knowing that the AEB will take over in case of emergencies, including those at low speed.

An example could be where a driver with no AEB installed would consciously reduce speed and be particularly alert when approaching a group of pedestrians on the footway. However, the driver may be less likely to pay attention knowing that if a pedestrian should unexpectedly step into the path of the car the AEB would stop the car faster than could she or he, the driver.

Current features of recorded use and reductions in collisions cited due to installation and use of AEB described and referenced in Chapter 9 are:

- 48%/42% reduction in pedestrians killed/seriously injured (Rosen et al. 2013)
- 27% – all potential accident savings (Euro NCAP 2014)

> In view of the foregoing, the judgemental percentage assumed for accident reduction scenarios of AEB, *the 'what if' percentage reduction assumed for the AEB implementation scenario is 30%, thereby reducing the basic value to 70% of its projected amount.*

Improved Vehicle Design

Unlike EDR and AEB, the reduction of pedestrian collision severity results from improved vehicle design irrespective of the driver's physical and mental condition and attitude to driving. The severity of any collision between a vehicle and a pedestrian will depend on the vehicle's speed and configuration and the exact position and physical characteristics of the pedestrian.

Current features of recorded use and reductions in collisions cited due to improved vehicle design described and referenced in Chapter 10 are:

- 38%/10% – average- vs low-performing cars – Strandroth et al. 2011. These results applied to urban areas with speed limits up to 50 km/h (approximately 30 mph), although no significant reduction was found in higher speed zones (DaCoTA 2012)
- 6% fatalities, 9% seriously injured pedestrians on German roads – 22 Euro NCAP point score (Euro NCAP 2012)

> In view of the foregoing, *the percentage assumed for pedestrian casualty reduction for improved vehicle design is 10%, thereby reducing the basic value to 90% of its projected amount.*

Casualty Reduction Scenario

As indicated earlier, trends based on general improvements (Mitchell and Allsop 2013) provide basic values of casualties to which the 'what if' percentage casualty reductions detailed above are applied. These basic values for seriously injured vary between approximately 2,000 and 3,000, depending on the assumptions for calculation. Because pedestrian fatalities are approximately 12% of those seriously injured, the respective values of killed or seriously injured (KSI) are increased here by this 12% to 2,240 and 3,360 for the year 2030. Figure 12.1 shows the area of trends and the values quoted.

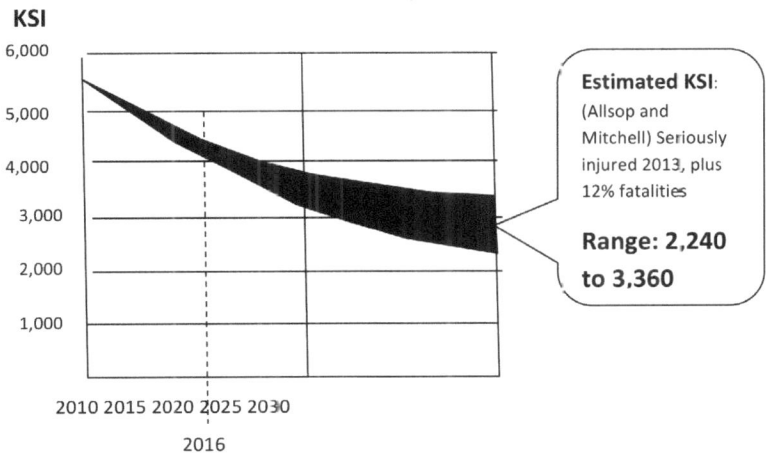

Figure 12.1 Forecast KSI, pedestrians, to year 2030 (Source: Mitchell and Allsop 2013, Figure 8, for seriously injured pedestrians, plus estimated 12% fatalities)

A summary of the reductions through to the estimated casualty numbers on the estimated scenario for the year 2030 is shown in Table 12.1 below. The various numbered columns (nos. 1 to 10) of the table show:

1. Method of potential reductions, i.e. EDR, AEB and improved vehicle design.
2. Range of reductions described in the various chapters on each method and summarised in the descriptions of the rationale for the reductions above.
3. Assumed scenario reduction percentage for each of the methods, based on judgemental, conservative 'what if' values. Each of the values reflects the percentage reduction in the populations for which the evidential reductions were achieved, and assumes that a future total population would experience a similar percentage reduction.
4. Combined percentages reduction of Column 3 to a single percentage for application to year 2030. Total reduced percentage: = 80% x 70% x 90% = 50.4% = 50% rounded

5. Estimated year 2030 killed, based on trends as stated in Mitchell and Allsop (2013) that the projected casualties for seriously injured vary between approximately 2,000 and 3,000, depending on the assumptions for calculation. Assumed further pedestrians killed are approximately 12% of those seriously injured, i.e. 240 and 360 respectively.
6. Estimated year 2030 seriously injured, as used for Item No. 3, above.
7. Estimated year 2030 slightly injured, based on proportion of slightly injured to KSI trends in year 2015 on the same basis as used for Item No. 3, above.
8. Estimated year 2030 killed, based on scenario estimation – high and low estimates increased by percentage of Item 4.
9. Estimated year 2030 seriously injured, based on scenario estimation – high and low estimates, increased by percentage of Item 4.
10. Estimated year 2030 slightly injured, based on scenario estimation – high and low estimates, increased by percentage of Item 4.

METHOD OF REDUCTION (1)	CITED REDUCTION RANGE % (2)	ASSUMED SCENARIO REDUCTION % (3)	REDUCED PERCENTAGE OF MITCHELL AND ALLSOP PROJECTIONS (4)	EXISTING ESTIMATED CASUALTY NUMBER RANGE FOR YEAR 2030 (Mitchell and Allsop 2013) with slightly injured estimated separately			ESTIMATED FUTURE NUMBER RANGE (rounded) including full-scale implementation of black box, AEB and improved vehicle design		
				Killed (5)	Severe Injury (6)	Slight Injury (7)	Killed (8)	Severe Injury (9)	Slight Injury (10)
EDR	18 - 60	20	50% rounded	240	2,000	8,000	120	1,000	4,000
AEB	48 - 27	30		360	3,000	12,000	180	1,500	6,000
Improved vehicle design	38 - 6	10							

Table 12.1 Casualty reduction scenario summary

The results of the scenario of implementing full EDR, AEB and improved vehicle design compared to the year 2013 casualties and those indicated by trends resulting from general road and traffic improvements are summarised in Table 12.2. The numbers shown indicate an approximate halving of the 2013 numbers if continuing trends continue to the year 2030. A further halving by the year 2030 if the scenario envisaging implementation of the black box, AEB and vehicle design improvement is mandated, based on available evidence.

SEVERITY BASIS	KILLED	SEVERELY INJURED	KSI	SLIGHTLY INJURED
2013 Actual (DfT 2014)	398	4,998	5,396	18,637
2030 Estimate: trends – general road and traffic improvements (Mitchell and Allsop 2013)	240 – 360 (Assumed for calculation purposes in this estimation)	2,000 – 3,000	2,240 – 3,360	8,000 to 12,000 (Assumed for calculation purposes in this estimation)
2030 Scenario: trends, above, with black box, AEB and vehicle design improvement	120 – 180	1,000 – 1,500	1,120 – 1,680	3,900 – 5,850

Table 12.2 Summary comparison actual and estimated pedestrian casualties

The results of the scenario are shown graphically in Figure 12.2. This shows the selected area of the trends for KSI under the selected scenario compared to those shown earlier in Figure 12.1 The trends are shown as a slight curve, reflecting a rate of decrease similar to that for the trends forecast for the basic values. This would respond to implementation of changes as new vehicles are introduced into the nation's fleet, with a potential period of about 15 years to 2030.

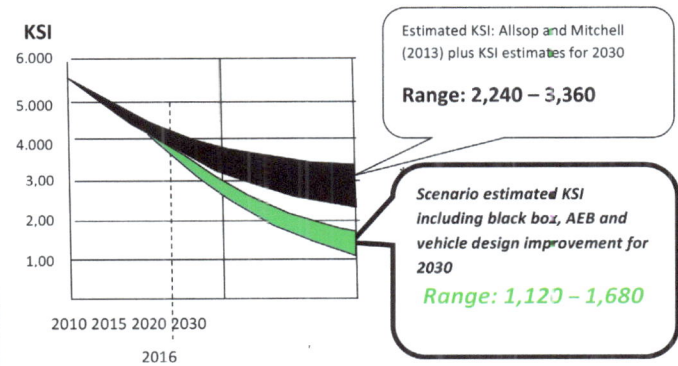

Figure 12.2 Potential KSI reduction scenario comparison. Values for year 2030 as per Table 12.2

★

> This chapter has undertaken the informative exercise of estimating, approximately and based on a specific scenario of implementing key technological improvements, likely future pedestrian casualties. The bases for these estimates are results of studies which have shown considerable evidence of reduced collisions of all types, a significant proportion of which involve pedestrians. *Yet the scenario estimates, which show a potential reduction of nearly 70% over existing estimates to the year 2030, still show at least 120 people killed, nearly 1,000 severely injured and nearly 4,000 slightly injured annually. As more studies and, hopefully, practical trials leading to mandated changes to the vehicle fleet and driver abilities lead to anticipated pedestrian casualty reductions, perhaps the conservative values assumed for the scenario can be revised downwards. Also, emerging factors such as increased driver and pedestrian distraction due to electronic devices must be considered. The challenge will be to generate enough public awareness and indignation to demand that elected officials and professional staff at local, regional and national level implement the necessary legislation to bring about these improvements.* The universe of pedestrians and the many benefits that will result deserve nothing less.

References

Department for Transport (2014) *Reported Road Casualties Great Britain* 2014. London.

Mitchell, C.G.B and R.E. Allsop (2013) *Projections of Road Casualties in Great Britain to 2030, for PACTS*, March 2013. London.

Schoon, John G. (2015) *Estimated Pedestrian Casualty Levels for 2030 Based on EDR, AEB and Vehicle Design Improvements*. Draft unpublished working paper.

END NOTE

During the nearly two years production of this book many aspects of road traffic and pedestrian safety have evolved. Yet the number of pedestrian casualties since 2015 in Britain has not changed significantly, remaining at over 5,000 KSI annually.

Development of electric and 'self drive' vehicles is continuing by several existing and new manufacturers. The need for recognition of objects to be avoided during the trajectory of such vehicles, including pedestrians in their varied configurations and circumstances, remains a considerable challenge. Nevertheless, progress is being made and more manufacturers are offering 'safety packages' which address driver monitoring, Automated Emergency Braking (AEB) and improved vehicle design to reduce injuries in the case of collisions.

Yet these technological advances are still provided mostly on 'luxury' vehicles. There is no significant movement by government to impose regulations on the fleet in general. Neither is there any movement even to equip governmental vehicles with such safety packages. Due to the imposition of strict seat-belt requirements in vehicles the number and severity of occupants' injuries fell dramatically. Similar legislation to avoid and mitigate the severity of pedestrian/vehicle collisions is urgently needed.

In addition to technological advances, little progress has been made in the last two years to address basic geometric road crossing designs. Designs are needed which accommodate the millions of people who are unable to walk safely because their abilities to cross the road do not fit current design norms. Health, welfare and, importantly also, economic implications of such lack of mobility, have not been successfully quantified. Such concerns require urgent attention.

Lightning Source UK Ltd.
Milton Keynes UK
UKHW051437160819
348057UK00001BA/10/P